ULTRAMICRO METHODS

FOR CLINICAL LABORATORIES

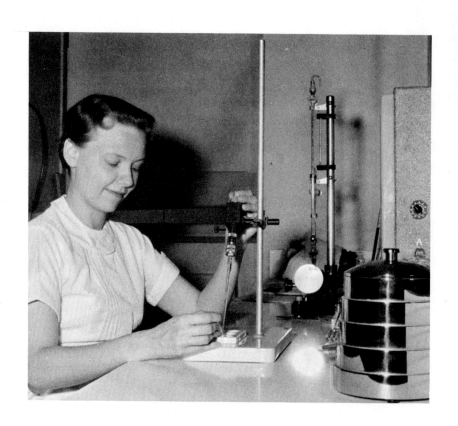

ULTRAMICRO METHODS

FOR CLINICAL LABORATORIES

———————————— SECOND EDITION ————————————

Edwin M. Knights, Jr., M.D.
Director of Pathology Department,
Providence Hospital, Detroit, Michigan

Roderick P. MacDonald, Ph.D.
Director of Clinical Chemistry,
Harper Hospital, Detroit, Michigan

Jaan Ploompuu
Research Associate in Ultramicro Chemistry,
Hurley Hospital, Flint, Michigan

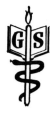

GRUNE & STRATTON 1962
NEW YORK   LONDON

Library of Congress Catalog Card No. 56-12594

Copyright 1962
Grune & Stratton, Inc.
381 Park Avenue South
New York 16, N.Y.

Printed and bound in U.S.A. (U-B)

RB
40
K71u
1962
Locked
Case

CONTENTS

v

149343

Foreword

The employment of accurate and rapid ultramicro methods for quantitative determination of chemical constituents of blood or other body fluid represents an important advance in the clinical laboratory.

The need for such methods is readily recognized whenever only minute amounts of material are available, as in infants, children and small experimental animals; whenever superficial veins are not accessible, available, or adequate for withdrawal of blood; or when frequent sampling or multiple testing of blood is desired, even in adults with large and easily accessible superficial veins.

Until now these methods have been employed mainly in larger clinical laboratories or in biologic experimental studies, inasmuch as an extra measure of skill and care is necessary. Compared with the grosser methods, the performance of ultramicro technics requires less space and permits economy of equipment and reagents. Clinically, their employment in selected patients has been advantageous to the patients and has regularly proved popular with the attending physicians. Ultramicro chemical methods are now a valuable adjunct to modern clinical pathology.

In presenting this manual on "Ultramicro Methods for Clinical Laboratories," the authors have rendered a distinct service to clinical pathology, making available in ready form a number of practical technics. In view of the constant development of new and refined methods in this field, one can confidently expect frequent and repeated revisions and additions in subsequent editions of this work.

S. E. GOULD, M.D.
Professor of Pathology
Wayne University
College of Medicine

Preface To The Second Edition

The growth of ultramicro chemistry has proceeded at such a pace that it is quite astounding to realize that our first edition, published but five years ago, was the first such book to be written specifically on the utilization of ultramicro methods in the clinical laboratory. The enthusiastic acceptance of ultramicro methods of analysis during the brief period has been most rewarding to our faith in them. The increased size of this book is testimony to the numerous innovations which have appeared, and indeed improvements are occurring at such a rate that it is a challenge to keep abreast of them.

Many laboratories have adopted those ultramicro technics peculiar to their needs, while others have seen fit to develop complete ultramicro divisions. The unitized concept of ultramicro testing, as developed by Sanz and introduced by Beckman/Spinco, represents another phase in the simplification of procedures. The development of a moderately-priced spectro-colorimeter by Beckman/ Spinco and the adaptation of the Coleman Junior spectro-photometer to ultramicro work reduces the cost of installing these methods significantly, and, as a result, large numbers of laboratories are either performing them now or intend to do so in the near future.

It is well to remember, however, that the basic principles of ultramicro chemistry are just as valid as when they were first enumerated. Proper training of the technologist and careful laboratory work are just as important as before. A fact that has already become painfully apparent is that the substitution of "gimmicks" for methods that have proven their reliability throughout prolonged clinical use is rarely successful. Furthermore, a careful survey of available equipment described in this book will demonstrate that the most expensive or complicated apparatus available is not necessarily either the most suitable or the most dependable.

We are grateful, nonetheless, to the manufacturers who have spent so much time and money to offer new ingenious equipment for ultramicro chemical analysis; a great service has been rendered to the scientific practice of medicine. It is to be hoped, also, that various scientific organizations will continue to present opportunities for interested persons to acquaint themselves with the newer equipment by sponsoring more workshops and discussions of this rapidly-growing adjunct to clinical medicine.

We wish to acknowledge the most valuable assistance of many of our associates in the preparation of this book; in particular we are indebted to Dr. James S. Brush for his work on the Corinth calcium method, to Dr. G. Thomas Passananti for his contributions to the chapters on flame photometry and pH, to Mr. James L. Whitehouse for his assistance in evaluating and comparing equipment, to Mr. John Bugbee, Mr. Royal Le Fave, Mrs. Thomasine Lewis and Mrs. Frances McCormick. We also wish to thank the equipment manufacturers who have provided many of the photographs which appear in this book.

THE AUTHORS

Preface to the First Edition

The increased use of hospital laboratories in diagnosis of human disease has been little short of phenomenal. Today's medical school graduates, trained in the value of maintaining proper electrolyte balance and familiar with recent innovations in clinical pathology, have placed an unprecedented demand on laboratory facilities. Meanwhile, hospital laboratories have made continual progress in devising and improving methods to supply the clinician with accurate blood chemistry results. The history of clinical biochemistry has been one of continual progress with modification superimposed upon modification.

All of this interest in blood chemistry has resulted in greater amounts of blood being removed from the sick patient. This has caused considerable concern to many who feel the leech has been abandoned only to be replaced by the medical technologist. There should be some method to improve the situation other than by purchasing larger sized syringes. The problem becomes particularly acute in those cases involving immature infants, extremely obese patients, third-degree burn cases, or patients requiring intravenous feeding. Here it would be particularly desirable to obtain blood by a method other than venipuncture, since it is often necessary to perform determinations on relatively small amounts of blood.

The analysis of blood samples smaller than those usually available for routine technics has usually been approached by attempts to use "cut down" versions of macromethods of analysis. The disadvantages of this approach, whether by titrimetric, colorimetric or gasometric methods are quite apparent. The apparatus and procedures of the tests have been designed for larger aliquots; reducing the sample size often tends to introduce considerable chance of error. Usually the original examination has been prepared so as to give a reading in the optimal titrimetric or spectrophotometric range and deviation from this range may greatly decrease the sensitivity and accuracy. Often the amount of blood required still necessitates a venipuncture. An alternative approach to this problem is the use of *ultramicro* methods of analysis. There is no exact definition of *ultramicro*, but it is generally considered to include determinations of micrograms (0.001 mg.) or microliters (0.001 ml.), sometimes referred to as *gammas* and *lambdas*. As the individual test requires only 0.01 to 0.03 ml. of serum, a fairly complete survey can be performed on 0.2 to 0.3 ml. of blood obtained by pricking the heel or finger. The methods are also particularly well adapted to the examination of small quantities of cerebrospinal fluid.

Microgram analytical methods have already made significant contributions to such diversified fields as enzyme histochemistry, tissue cultures, and protozoology but it is only recently that very extensive clinical use has been made of them. Such investigators as Rappaport, Glick, Natelson, Kirk, and Caraway have done much to further our knowledge of their clinical usage. Gradually more and more hospitals are adopting ultramicro methods as a solution to their problems, and as their interest in the technic grows, the need for a practical manual of methods for hospital use becomes more acute. It is sincerely hoped that this book will fill that need. As Otto Schales said in his presidential address to the Seventh Annual Meeting of the American Association of Clinical Chemists, "All of us have encountered the dilemma of a battery of tests to be done with insufficient blood. Ultramicro methods will be of great value in such instances."

Unfortunately inadequate knowledge of ultramicro methods combined with excessive demands on already existing facilities and personnel in hospital chemistry departments has resulted in their rather slow acceptance. Actually, once the ultramicro division has been established it proves itself remarkably adaptable to routine use and results can be obtained with an accuracy that compares favorably with standard procedure. But in order to achieve such accuracy, samples should be obtained and analyzed by competent technologists trained in this subspecialty. As the equipment, reagents and glassware are used only by the ultramicro chemist, they should be his personal responsibility and kept exclusively for his use. Ultramicro chemistry has a distinct advantage in the minimum amount of space required for its operation; however, it is very desirable that it be kept as separate as possible from the frenzied activity of the routine hospital chemistry department. Once in operation it proves extremely valuable, not only in the analysis of blood specimens from the previously mentioned types of patients but also in providing a convenient means of checking questionable results obtained with macromethods where only a small amount of serum is still available. The potentialities of the ultramicro method in research have barely been explored. When combined with the use of microhematocrit methods, it is extremely useful in the management of difficult pediatric cases. It can also be expanded to include the fields of paper chromatography and paper electrophoresis. Such laboratory tests as non-protein nitrogen, urea nitrogen, total protein, creatinine, albumin, glucose, sodium, potassium, chloride, icteric index, bilirubin, cholesterol, thymol turbidity, cephalin flocculation, phosphatase, amylase and carbon dioxide combining power have proved adaptable to ultramicro methods and provide a well-rounded selection for the practicing physician.

THE AUTHORS

1

Setting Up Ultramicro Chemistry in the General Laboratory

In the general hospital laboratory, an ultramicro division may be established as a subdivision of the chemistry department, but it is best to keep it quite separate physically from routine chemical procedures. At Harper Hospital, ultramicro chemical methods and research had been used for many years, but attempts to incorporate them into the hospital routine were unsuccessful until a separate subdivision had been properly organized and equipped. As the ultramicro chemist must work as quietly and with as little disturbance as possible, he should be separated from the routine macrochemical procedures. A sink with a suction attachment and a handy reagent shelf are important. A "lazy Susan" type of dispenser with one or more levels is useful in putting all of the necessary reagents at the technologist's fingertips without necessitating his leaving his seat.

Since the equipment, reagents, and glassware are used only by the ultramicro technologist, they should be kept exclusively for his or her use. A possible exception to this is the flame photometer on which the sodium and potassium determinations are performed. The technologist must be completely responsible for the glassware and its maintenance. Results can be obtained with an accuracy comparable to standard procedures, but in order to achieve this, samples should be obtained and analyzed by competent technologists who have received additional instructions in this subspecialty.

A small group of selected reference books and pertinent articles will always be of considerable value for consultation and these should be located conveniently in the laboratory for the use of the ultramicro technologist. We have included here a list of reference works that form a small "library" of useful and important information.

Books on Methodology
BIER, M.: Electrophoresis: Theory, Methods, and Applications. New York, Academic Press, 1959.
BLOCK, R. J., DURRUM, E. L., AND ZWEIG, G.: Paper Chromatography and Paper Electrophoresis. 2nd Ed. New York, Academic Press, 1958.

1

CARAWAY, W. T.: Microchemical Methods for Blood Analysis. Springfield, Ill., Charles C Thomas, 1960.

CONWAY, E. J.: Micro Diffusion Analysis and Volumetric Error. 4th Ed. New York, MacMillan Co., 1958.

COUNCIL ON CLINICAL CHEMISTRY: Workshops on Microchemistry, Pre-Workshop and Workshop Manuals. Chicago, American Society of Clinical Pathologists, 1960.

KING, E. J., AND WOTTON, I. D. P.: Micro-Analysis in Medical Biochemistry. 3rd Ed. New York, Grune & Stratton, 1956.

KIRK, P. L.: Quantitative Ultramicroanalysis. New York, Wiley & Sons, 1951.

MATTENHEIMER, H.: Mikromethoden für das Klinisch-Chemische und Biochemische Laboratorium. Berlin, Walter de Gruyter & Co., 1961.

MEITES, S., AND FAULKNER, W. R.: Manual of Practical Micro and General Procedures in Clinical Chemistry. Springfield, Ill., Charles C Thomas, 1962.

MILTON, R. F., AND WATERS, W. A.: Methods of Quantitative Microanalysis. 2nd Ed. New York, St. Martin's Press, 1955.

NATELSON, S.: Microtechniques of Clinical Chemistry. Springfield, Ill., Charles C Thomas, 1957.

RAPPAPORT, F.: Rapid Microchemical Methods for Blood and CSF Examinations. New York, Grune & Stratton, 1949.

REINER, M.: Standard Methods of Clinical Chemistry. Vol. I. New York, Academic Press, 1953.

SELIGSON, D.: Standard Methods of Clinical Chemistry. Vol. II. New York, Academic Press, 1958.

TELOH, H. A.: Clinical Flame Photometry. Springfield, Ill., Charles C Thomas, 1959.

WILKINSON, R. H.: Chemical Micromethods in Clinical Medicine. Springfield, Ill., Charles C Thomas, 1960.

WOLSTENHOLME, G. E. W., AND MILLAR, E. C. P.: Ciba Foundation Symposium on Paper Electrophoresis. Boston, Little, Brown & Co., 1956.

Articles on Methodology

CARAWAY, W. T., AND FANGER, H.: Ultramicro procedures in clinical chemistry. *Am. J. Clin. Path. 25:* 317-331, 1955.

GAMBINO, S. R.: Variation of plasma pH with temperature of separation; Heparinized vacuum tubes for determination of plasma pH, plasma CO_2 content, and blood oxygen saturation; Normal values for adult human venous plasma pH and CO_2 content; Comparisons of pH in human arterial, venous and capillary blood; the Clinical value of routine determinations of venous plasma pH in acid-base problems. *Am. J. Clin. Path. 32:* 270-272, 285-308, 1959.

HOLADAY, D. A., AND VEROSKY, M.: Improved micromanometric methods for the analysis of respiratory gases in plasma and whole blood. *J. Lab. & Clin. Med. 47:* 634-644, 1956.

KAPLAN, S. A., AND DEL CARMEN, F. T.: Quantitative ultramicro-analysis for the clinical laboratory. *Pediatrics 17:* 857-869, 1956.

KAPLAN, S. A., YUCEOGLU, A. M., AND STRAUSS, J.: Chemical microanalysis: Analysis of capillary and venous blood. *Pediatrics 24:* 270-274, 1959.

KNIGHTS, E. M., JR., MACDONALD, R. P., AND PLOOMPUU, J.: An improved ultramicro pipet. *Am. J. Clin. Path. 30:* 91-92, 1958.

KNIGHTS, E. M., JR.: Ultramicroanalytic methods now adaptable to hospital use. *J.A.M.A. 166:* 1175-1176, 1958.

NATELSON, S.: Routine use of ultramicromethods in the clinical laboratory. *Am J. Clin. Path. 21:* 1153-1172, 1951.

O'Brien, D., Ibbott, F., and Pinfield, A.: Critical evaluation of a new ultramicro system for routine clinical chemistry procedures. *Clin. Chem. 7:* 521-535, 1961.

Sanz, M. C.: Ultramicro methods and standardization of equipment. *Clin. Chem. 3:* 406-419, 1957.

Sobel, A. E. and Hanok, A.: Ultramicro quantitative analysis in clinical laboratories. *Mikrochemie 39:* 51-68, 1952

van Haga, P. Reinouts, and de Wael, J.: Ultramicro Methods. Advances in Clinical Chemistry, Vol. 4. New York, Academic Press, 1961, pp. 321-350.

Choosing the Method

The selection of an analytical procedure for adaptation to an ultramicro technic requires very careful consideration. Many methods may simply be scaled down into the ultramicro range, others simply will not work when this approach is followed. The common procedures of inorganic phosphate by Fiske and Subbarow and calcium by Clark and Collip are examples of the latter. The rationale is usually lack of sensitivity, but other factors certainly are involved. The tedious but certain trial-and-error approach will determine if scaling down may be used.

Most colorimetric methods have a high degree of sensitivity and relative specificity. The selection of the proper instrument for measuring this color usually determines how much of this sensitivity may be utilized. If we assume the instrument is ideal, maximum precision is obtained at optical density 0.434 (36.8 per cent transmission) with the error of measurement increasing rapidly below 10 per cent and above 85 per cent transmission. If we wished to make use of a method at maximum precision (O.D. 0.434), the smaller the diameter (or total volume) and the higher the extinction coefficient,* the less substance would be required to give the desired result. For example[19] (*see* Table 1), using a cuvet 32 mm. in diameter, with a color whose specific extinction coefficient is about 50, 639 μg. of a colored substance is required to produce the same light absorbance as 0.0065 μg. would produce in a tube 2 mm. in diameter when its specific extinction coefficient is about 20,000. Assuming the extinction coefficient could not be altered through a modification of the method (for example, by decreasing the dilution of the chromogen), narrowing the diameter of the tube from only 8 mm. to 2 mm. would reduce the volume required from 500 to 30 lambdas and in the case of a substance whose extinction coefficient is 1000, reduce the required amount of constituent from 2.17 to 0.13 μg. This is achieved without sacrificing the 10 mm. length of light path by reducing the

---

* Extinction coefficient: The absorbance (or optical density) of a 1 per cent solution in a 10 mm. light path. This value is most useful in comparing the sensitivity of two colorimetric methods. In practice, a different concentration and length of light path is often used. Consult a standard text in analytical chemistry for this conversion.

TABLE 1.—SIZE OF SAMPLE AS A FUNCTION OF DIAMETER AND EXTINCTION COEFFICIENT
IN COLORIMETRIC METHODS[19]

Diameter	Vol./10 mm. Length	$\mu g.$ Constituent for O.D. 0.434 (36. 8% T) 1% when $E_{1cm.}$ is		
mm.		50	1000	20,000
32	8050	638.74	34.94	1.947
8	500	43.40	2.17	0.109
2	30	2.60	0.13	0.0065

lateral dimension of the cuvet. The 10 mm. light path should be considered
essential, and should not be sacrificed to obtain a smaller volume.

Laboratory Control

Several preliminary investigations should be performed before any ultramicro procedure is adopted for routine use in the laboratory.

1. The ultramicro and macro technics to be used should be performed simultaneously on a venous blood specimen. It is advantageous if the two results are
comparable in a laboratory in which both technics are to be used. If necessary,
ultramicro procedures should be calibrated using specimens analyzed by
macro methods, as is required in the case of icterus index. If the results of
both methods agree, determinations on patients may be alternated between the
two procedures when necessary. Ultramicro methods may also be used to
check macro methods when the quantity of specimen precludes a check by the
macro method. Another advantage of having both methods agree is the ability
of the laboratory to use an ultramicro method if the quantity of specimen
received is not sufficient for a macro determination. All these alternatives may
be used in the laboratory without influencing the final result, which would
require an explanation to the physician ordering the test.

2. The ultramicro methods using capillary blood should be compared with
macro procedures performed on venous blood obtained from the same patient
at the same time (*see* discussion on normal values).

3. Whole blood macro technics should be compared with capillary serum
ultramicro technics if serum is to be substituted for whole blood.

4. Controls consisting of samples of known value should be run con-
comitantly.

The problem of laboratory control is best approached by reference to three
terms; accuracy, precision and reliability.[9] These terms are often used
interchangeably, but their meanings are quite different. Each represents a
different aspect of determining the quality of laboratory values.

Accuracy consists of comparing an observed result with the actual known value of the constituent under analysis. Often good accuracy is beyond the ability of a particular method to produce and may even be unnecessary. Many clinically useful methods fall short in accuracy, e.g., some glucose, uric acid, cholesterol, creatinine and other methods. Enzyme determinations in which rate of activity is expressed in somewhat arbitary units almost preclude good accuracy. So long as the expressed value of the result of the determination is a clinically significant representation of the particular substance, the method may be considered valid. However, the analyst should be aware of the lack of accuracy in a test and be alert to detect those situations when this may become significant.

Precision is the degree of variation in the reproducibility of the method. This is determined by analyzing an aliquot of the same sample repeatedly over a period of time. The less variation found during this time, the greater the precision. This is a measurement which is quite easily obtained. A high degree of precision is necessary for every laboratory. Many laboratory variables enter into the precision of a method and most of these variables may be controlled by the analyst. However, it follows that the greater the number of variables, the more difficult to control precision.[14] Some methods permit a higher degree of precision than others; the most satisfactory technic is usually the one that is simplest and most direct but which still gives adequate precision.

Reliability of a method is the ability to maintain accuracy and precision on a day-by-day basis in the laboratory. When accuracy and precision have been determined, then periodic checking serves to ascertain whether or not the test is performing as predicted.

It is usually desirable to determine the degree of precision required from a test. Many laboratories use as a "rule of thumb" an allowable error of 5 per cent. This may be satisfactory for some tests, but not for others. Certainly, a serum sodium level report of 140 ± 7 mEq./L. would disenchant any clinician. On the other hand, a value for allowable error might be satisfactory for use in one situation but not another, e.g., a greater precision is required for calcium in diagnosing hyperparathyroidism than in most other diseases.

If the method under consideration shows less precision than that required, various solutions are possible:

(1) One may, of course, resort to another method.

(2) Better control of all variables, including technic, units for measurement, instrumentation, etc.

(3) Replication may decrease error. The improvement in error by running a sample in duplicate, triplicate, etc. may be calculated.[9] If E is the observed confidence limit or error for a single determination, and E_x the maximum error permitted, then the number of replicates, N, necessary to achieve this is

$\left(\dfrac{E}{E_x} \right)^2$, or, transposing this, $E_x = \dfrac{E}{\sqrt{N}}$. For example, if the error of a method was found to be eight per cent when no greater than five per cent would be tolerated, then:

$$\text{Single determination } E_x = \frac{8}{\sqrt{1}} = 8 \text{ per cent}$$

$$\text{Duplicate} \qquad E_x = \frac{8}{\sqrt{2}} = 5.7 \text{ per cent}$$

$$\text{Triplicate} \qquad E_x = \frac{8}{\sqrt{3}} = 4.7 \text{ per cent}$$

Therefore, a triplicate analysis would be required to achieve the desired precision.

One caution should be noted, however. Higher precision should not be sought for purely esoteric reasons. Clinical significance should always be a determining factor.

Terms for Expressing Precision

Many people consider the use of statistics a sure route down the primrose path. Nonetheless, when we must analyze data in which a large number of individual events are involved, statistical analysis is the only positive (and possibly the only) approach. Out of the complexity of statistical mathematics we are evolving useful and practical applications.[8,17]

Copeland[6] has written regarding the confusion of terminology for expressing precision: "The problem of expressing laboratory precision is a maze of statistical terms and formulas which become entwined with problems of confidence and competence, often with a large emotional overlay. Everyone wants to do good work and to achieve a high degree of precision. However, unless we all proceed from the same reference point, no real progress can be made. Precision should not become a matter of "one-upmanship" based on the clever use of terminology."

Most workers today are agreed that standard deviation represents our best method for expressing precision. The term "standard deviation" is a measure of the dispersion of a group of values about their mean (or average). Two blood glucose determinations of 125 mg. per cent and 175 mg. per cent have a mean of 150 mg. per cent. The same mean is obtained from values of 148 and 152 mg. per cent. Obviously the latter represents a more satisfactory value; the two figures lie much closer to their mean. When a large series of measurements is involved, plus and minus one standard deviation unit includes 68 per cent of the measurements, plus and minus two standard deviation units includes 95 per cent, and plus and minus three standard deviation units includes 99.7 per cent.

Control Charts

A study by Belk and Sunderman in 1947[3] led many laboratory directors to consider the necessity of strict control of chemical methods. Levey and Jennings[16] first proposed a control chart, using pooled specimens of serum or plasma as standards. This technic has been developed by others[4,9,10] to the point where it offers a practical and simple method of determining laboratory precision and reproducibility.

A batch of pooled human serum is prepared by adding sufficient glucose and bilirubin to bring the levels of these constituents up to 100 mg. per cent and 2 mg. per cent respectively.[4] For ultramicro use, this serum is divided into individual samples of about 0.5 ml. each and placed in a deep-freeze until required. The individual specimen is thawed at about 30-35 C. on the day of use. At least 30 determinations on individual days are required to begin the statistical analysis. The standard deviation for each method is calculated from these data as follows:

$$\text{S.D.} = \sqrt{\frac{\Sigma(x - \overline{x})^2}{N - 1}}$$

S.D. = standard deviation
Σ = "sum of"
$\overline{x}$ = arithmetic mean of N determinations
x = a single determination
$x - \overline{x}$ = deviation of a single determination from the mean

To make standard deviation useful, "allowable error" is calculated from it and used for subsequent determinations.

$$\text{Allowable error (in per cent)} = \frac{3 \text{ S.D.}}{M} \times 100$$

S.D. = standard deviation
M = mean

A control chart is prepared for each determination with the analytical values (expressed in mg. per cent, mEq./L., etc.) as the ordinate and the date the test was performed as the abscissa. The mean obtained from the statistical study is drawn as a line parallel to the x-axis and parallel lines drawn to show the limits of allowable error.[9] Comparison of any subsequently determined value with the values on this chart will show whether or not the method is "in control."

A second method of preparing data for a control chart is to treat successive determinations as pairs.[9,10,20] The mean of each pair and the differences between each pair (the range, or R) are plotted on a control chart similar to the one described above. The 95 per cent confidence limit (the range in which a single value will fall 95 times out of 100) for the mean of a series of determinations is $\pm 1.88 \times (R)$, where the value R is obtained by averaging the range values, R. The confidence limit for the range is $3.27 \times (R)$. Only one limit need be considered, since the other limit is zero.

A somewhat simpler method for calculating standard deviation is the use of duplicates in routine analysis.[6] Ten routine analyses are run in duplicate. Find the difference between each set of the duplicate measurements (d), and square these differences (d^2). Add the squares of the differences between duplicates to get the sum, or Σd^2. Then

$$\text{Standard deviation} = \pm \sqrt{\frac{(\text{sum differences between duplicates})^2}{2 \ (\text{numbers of pairs})}}$$

Number of pairs $= n$

$$\text{S.D.} = \pm \sqrt{\frac{\Sigma d^2}{2n}}$$

To determine if the variation between runs is significantly greater than the variation within one run, Henry[10] suggested the use of duplicate standards. Duplicate analysis is performed daily on aliquots of the same sample for about 20 days. The mean of each pair (x) and the differences between each pair (the range, R) are plotted. Limits of 2 S.D. and 3 S.D. for x are $\pm$ 1.25 R and $\pm$ 1.88 R, respectively, where the value of R is obtained by averaging the range of values, R. The upper 2 S.D. and 3 S.D. limits for the range, R, are 2.18 R and 3.27 R respectively. When the R values are in control, this would indicate the variation between runs is significantly greater than that within runs.

The use of 95 per cent confidence limits (2 S.D. units) would seem to be most appropriate. In other words, that a single determination would have a given $\pm$ error within this range 95 times out of 100. In practice it is often obvious that these limits are too great, and the desired precision falls within the range of $\pm$ 1 S.D. unit. It is best to judge acceptable limits only after calculations have been made, and with the desirable precision kept in mind. When standard deviation units of 2, or even 1, are used, it must be remembered that out of limit results may be obtained without demonstrable cause, and one is setting up higher standards of precision than would ordinarily be obtained from the method.

There is a tendency among those laboratory directors who use control charts to keep them as personal information. It is probably best to keep them in open view in the laboratory. Technologists then become control conscious and interested in upgrading the quality of their work. There is always a danger of prejudicial handling of control specimens, but education helps to eliminate this problem.

Other more elegant and often useful statistical calculations are available for use in laboratory control. These include the "t" test, analysis of variance, the "F" ratio, sequential analysis, sensitivity analysis, and others. Many good statistical texts are available for reference on the use of these determinations.

Laboratory Error

Benenson et al.[4] list the following common factors causing a method to go out of control: deteriorated or faulty reagents, variable laboratory conditions, careless technic, and poorly trained or inexperienced personnel. One insidious source of error in the laboratory is the presence of free residual chlorine in distilled water. In tap water, free chlorine is in equilibrium with hydrochloric and hypochlorous acid. Chlorine is volatilized in the distillation process and both chlorine and hypochlorous acid may appear in the distillate.

Caraway[5] found chlorine present in distilled water in concentrations up to 1 p.p.m. (1 μg. per ml.) In the analysis of bilirubin by the method of Evelyn and Malloy, chlorine-contaminated water resulted in a 12 per cent decrease in optical density. Titration of chloride by mercuric nitrate was not affected by the small amount of chloride present in the chlorine-contaminated water. Chlorine-contaminated distilled water did not affect results in the determination of phosphate (Fiske-Subbarow method), glucose (Benedict method), protein (Biuret method) and ammonia nitrogen (nesslerization).

The following test is recommended for determining the presence of free chlorine in distilled water:[5]

Test reagent: 0.1 Gm. O-tolidine dihydrochloride in 100 ml. 1 N hydrochloric acid. Solution is stable and should be colorless.

Test: Add 1.0 ml. reagent to 100 ml. of water, mix thoroughly, and note color at the end of 5 minutes.

Test results: Yellow color is presumptive evidence for the presence of free chlorine. The test measures total available chlorine, regardless of the form in which it is present in water. A set of standards for semi-quantitative visual comparison may be prepared from potassium dichromate and cupric sulfate.[18]

Variations in the pH of clinical samples may be a source of error in enzyme determinations.[11] Variations in the pH of body fluids occur even when they are fresh. For example, blood may vary from about pH 7 to pH 7.8, and urine pH from 4.6 to 8. Samples of blood, serum and urine exposed to air lose CO_2 and an increase in pH will occur. The rapidity of this pH increase is dependent on such variables as volume of fluid, surface area and amount of agitation of the fluid during storage. When less sample is taken for the test, as in the case of ultramicro procedures, final pH may vary from that of the corresponding macro technic. An active program of laboratory control will serve to detect any of these situations.

Reference standard solutions may be analyzed concurrently with any unknown specimen, and in most ultramicro methods this technic is suggested as a daily routine. It will be especially helpful in the determination of an unfamiliar end-point.

Two types of commercially prepared products are available. One consists of a pure standard solution of the substance to be analyzed, the other a serum with known analytical values for the constituents. The latter may either be "synthetic serum" or human lyophilized serum. It should be recalled that pure standard or control solutions usually are not carried throughout the entire procedure. Also, other substances may be present in human serum which will enhance or inhibit the color reaction of the test substance. This is true, for example, in the mercuric nitrate titration for chloride, when the presence or absence of protein alters the end-point. Therefore it is usually best to use serum as a control, and in certain cases as a standard.

1. Lab-Trol (Dade Reagents, Inc.). Available with constituents in either the normal or pathologic range. This is a synthetic liquid, and is recommended for use in ultramicro work since the solution is stable and only very small quantities are used at one time.

2. Hyland Clinical Chemistry Control Serum (Hyland Laboratories, Los Angeles, Calif.). Available with constituents in either the normal or pathologic range. Must be reconstituted with distilled water. The solution is stable for 5 days (except for glucose) if stored under refrigeration (2 to 5 C.). Contains cholesterol. This serum has been analyzed by commonly used procedures, and the results reported.

3. Versatol (Warner-Chilcott Laboratories). Available with constituents in either the normal or pathologic range. Various constituents are removed from serum, then added in known quantities.[15] Must be reconstituted with distilled water. When reconstituted, glucose and bilirubin are stable for 2 days, the other constituents for one week.

4. Clinical Pathology Standards (College of American Pathologists). Separate ampules containing pure solutions of known amounts of glucose, nitrogen, chloride, calcium, uric acid, creatinine, phosphate, sodium and potassium.

(These and other products mentioned throughout the book may be obtained from the firms listed. The addresses of these suppliers have been placed conveniently in the Directory of Distributors and Producers, pp. 209-210.

Use of Factors

Calculations in this book often refer to the use of a "factor." This is derived from the equation:

$$\frac{OD\ unk}{OD\ std} \times Conc.\ std. = Conc.\ unk \tag{1}$$

or:

$$OD\ unk \times \frac{Conc.\ std.}{O.D.\ std.} = Conc.\ unk \tag{2}$$

$$a \qquad\qquad b$$

Expression *b* in the second equation is constant for a given series of analyses and is referred to as the "factor." The final calculation is thereby reduced to a single multiplication step. In the calibration procedure this factor is determined for a range of levels and the average is used *unless* there is a marked deviation at either high or low concentrations. In this case a calibration chart should be used. The use of a factor is valid only when the color produced conforms to Beer's law and consequently this relationship must be predetermined in the calibration procedure. Standards and control specimens should be used periodically to validate the precision of the method.

Normal Values

Probably no term in laboratory medicine is abused more than "normal value." If there is reservation toward this statement, the excellent book by Williams, *Biochemical Individuality*, should be studied.[21] The range from health to disease is a continuous spectrum; the black and white well defined, but numerous shades of gray between. No one is ever completely well or completely ill. It is these shades of gray that prove to be most troublesome. It would seem best to consider three ranges: definitely normal, definitely pathologic, and a zone of values which require still another laboratory or clinical approach. Nevertheless, we must continue to report normal values along with our results until these ideas are better recognized.

In the past many workers have reported normal values in standard deviation units based upon the arithmetic mean. Henry[12] has pointed out that biologic data frequently fall in a distribution based on the geometric rather than the arithmetic mean. These data are "normally" distributed only after log transformation, and the geometric mean is the antilog of the arithmetic mean of the logs of the observation. This type of distribution occurs when an arithmetic change in a cause makes a geometric change in effect. Thus the distribution must be normal for this type of calculation. This may be demonstrated in a histogram which will indicate if skewing is taking place. A range of values must be at least two-fold before a significant difference between a normal and a lognormal distribution appears. Skewing (or the tendency for more of the values to fall on one side of the mean than the other) is a factor which must be considered carefully in the analysis of normal values.

The use of percentiles in establishing normal values has been suggested by Herrera.[13] He points out that use of an extreme range is not desirable, since this method underestimates that 95 per cent range in small samples and overestimates it in large samples. Herrera believes that a narrower range than the 2.5 and 97.5 percentiles for healthy persons is desirable, and therefore recommends the 10th and 90th percentiles. To calculate the 10th percentile: (1) Order the observed analytical values from lowest to highest value, letting the lowest value be item No. 1, i.e., the item of rank 1. (2) To find which ordered item estimates the 10th percentile, multiple $(N + 1)$ by 10 per cent, where N is the sample size. $(N + 1)$ is used rather than N because it can be shown that this gives the better (unbiased) estimate of a percentile. If $N = 70$, then 10 per cent of 80 is 8.0, and the 8th ordered item is the estimate of the 10th percentile. If the result $0.10 \times (N + 1)$ is not a whole number, linear interpolation must be used between the values of the items actually obtained. It is best to avoid this situation by planning the sample size.

To estimate the 90th percentile, order the items from the highest to the lowest value, letting the highest value be item No. 1, and treat just as was done for the 10th percentile. Thus, in the example given above, the 90th percentile would be item No. 8 in the order from the highest to the lowest value. For calculations of the precision and variability of these percentile estimates, refer to the original article.

A persistent problem is the tendency to forget that children are not adults. Infants and children at various ages will vary in their biochemical constitution. For example, the hyperglycemic response of children to test doses of glucose varies with the age of the child.

The substitution of capillary blood for venous blood should also be given consideration in determining normal values. Blood from a cutaneous puncture has long been recognized to be essentially arterial blood. A glucose tolerance test performed simultaneously using capillary and venous blood will show a higher curve for the former than the latter.[7] The CO_2 of capillary serum is approximately 1 mEq./L. lower than venous serum, while the chloride of capillary serum is approximately 1 mEq./L. higher.[2]

Another factor to be considered in the analysis of normal values is the effect of eating on the results of the test. Annino[1] obtained blood from 32 apparently normal subjects and analyzed for urea nitrogen, glucose, carbon dioxide, chloride, sodium, potassium, creatinine, proteins, cholestrerol, calcium, phosphorus, and uric acid. Specimens were drawn before breakfast, and at 45 minutes and two hours after eating. At 45 minutes, glucose levels varied considerably, there was a small but significant drop in phosphorus and a small rise in sodium. With these exceptions there were no differences in results between the fasting specimen and the two post-prandial specimens.

There are other influences on the normal values of blood constituents which should be considered. For example, inorganic phosphate is somewhat higher in summer than in winter. Normal value ranges will ordinarily include this type of difference.

REFERENCES

1. ANNINO, J. S., AND RELMAN, A. S.: *Am. J. Clin. Path. 31:* 155, 1959.
2. ANRODE, H. G., AND McCRORY, W. W.: *Clin. Chem. 2:* 278, 1956.
3. BELK, W. P., AND SUNDERMAN, F. W.: *Am. J. Clin. Path. 17:* 853, 1947.
4. BENENSON, A. S., THOMPSON, H. L. AND KLUGERMAN, M. R.: *Am. J. Clin. Path. 25:* 575, 1955.
5. CARAWAY, W. T.: *Clin. Chem. 4:* 513, 1958.
6. COPELAND, B. E.: *Am. J. Clin. Path. 27:* 551, 1957
7. FOSTER, G. L.: *J. Biol. Chem. 55:* 291, 1923.
8. FREE, S. M., JR.: *Clin. Chem. 5:* 300, 1959.
9. HENRY, R. J., AND SEGALOVE, M.: *J. Clin. Path. 5:* 305, 1952.
10. HENRY, R. J.: *Clin. Chem. 5:* 309, 1959.
11. HENRY, R. J., AND CHIAMORI, N.: *Clin. Chem. 5:* 402, 1959.
12. HENRY, R. J.: *Am. J. Clin. Path. 34:* 326, 1960.
13. HERRERA, L.: *J. Lab. & Clin. Med. 52:* 34, 1958.
14. JOHNSON, E. A.: *Am. J. Med. Tech. 26:* 55, 1960.
15. KLEIN, B., AND WEISSMAN, M.: *Clin. Chem. 4:* 194, 1958.
16. LEVEY, S., AND JENNINGS, E. R.: *Am J. Clin. Path. 20:* 1059, 1950.
17. SELIGSON, D.: *Clin. Chem. 3:* 425, 1957.
18. SNELL, F. D., AND SNELL, C. T.: Colorimetric Methods of Analysis. Vol. II. Princeton, N. Y., D. Van Nostrand, 1949, p. 707.
19. SOBEL, A. E., AND HANOK, A.: *Mikrochemie, 39:* 51, 1952.
20. WERNIMONT, G.: *Indust. Eng. Chem., Anal. Ed. 18:* 587, 1946.
21. WILLIAMS, R. J.: *Biochemical Individuality,* New York, John Wiley and Sons, Inc., 1956.

2

Special Equipment

PIPETS

Choice of Pipets

The most significant factor in obtaining reproducibility of ultramicro methods is precision in pipetting the sample, standard, and reagents. Ultramicro pipets for measuring volumes of microliter proportions must be constructed with some type of automatic stopping point in order to obtain a precision of 1 per cent. The three types of ultramicro pipets, the constriction, overflow, and straight pipets (Fig. 1), are generally used in the clinical laboratory in one of two manners: either as *sample* or *reagent* pipets. Selection is largely a matter of personal preference and mechanical aptitude.

Ultramicro laboratories must also use one other type of pipet—the uncalibrated *transfer* pipet (Fig. 2). As its chief purpose is for filling the spectrophotometer microcells, it should be expressly designed for this purpose. All of the microcells must be filled with care from the bottom to avoid forming bubbles. A long glass pipet with a fine tip is adequate for filling the Bessey-Lowry cuvets used in the Beckman DU. Spinco and Coleman have provided special pipets for their ultramicro system. The original plastic Spinco transfer pipet was impossible to clean because of the sealed plastic end. This end should be cut off to permit flow-through cleaning, and a rubber bulb added to provide control over the pipetting. From the standpoint of potential sample contamination, the plastic joint near the tip of the Coleman transfer pipet is undesirable, but the soft plastic protects microcell surfaces (Fig. 3).

Straight Pipets

Simplest in construction are the capillary pipets or straight pipets; they are relatively inexpensive and can be constructed sturdily or built to meet special situations. For this reason they frequently have been used also as transfer pipets. Pipets of this design were described by Kirk and Craig,[1] and

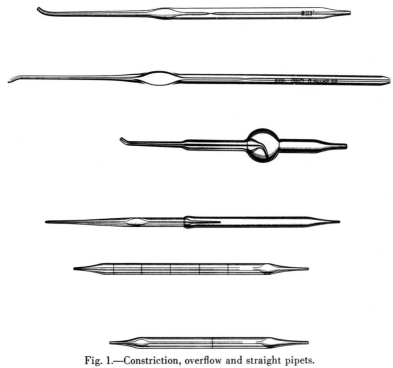

Fig. 1.—Constriction, overflow and straight pipets.

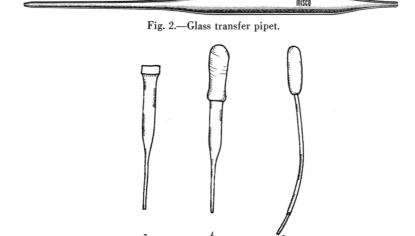

Fig. 2.—Glass transfer pipet.

Fig. 3.—Plastic Spinco transfer pipet (a) can be easily modified (b) by cutting off sealed end and adding rubber bulb for suction. Pipet may now be cleaned satisfactorily. The Coleman plastic transfer pipet (c) has a joint near the tip, which makes cleaning difficult.

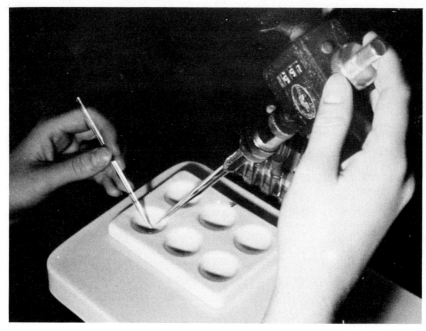

Fig. 4.—Straight pipet modified by Gilmont to make a pipet-buret.

by Sisco, Cunningham, and Kirk.[2]   They modified the basic capillary tube construction by adding two bulbs, one related to the contained volume and the other serving as a safety trap.

The straight pipet is commonly used together with some variety of pipet control—usually a glass hypodermic syringe of tuberculin type equipped with a flexible gasket for attachment to the pipet. Many modifications of both the pipets and the controls have been described;[3, 12, 17] more durable controls may be constructed entirely of metal. Elaborate controls have been developed, including mechanisms for semi-automatic or automatic delivery; these can transform the capillary pipet into a highly accurate capillary buret (Fig. 4).

Constriction Pipets

The conventional constriction pipet is made by heating a capillary tube until the tube partly collapses to form a sharp point of lesser internal diameter. In use, the liquid is drawn beyond the point of constriction and then blown forward gently. Increased resistance will be experienced as the meniscus reaches the constriction point. The tip is now wiped and the contents expelled by blowing slightly harder. Directions for constructing one version of this

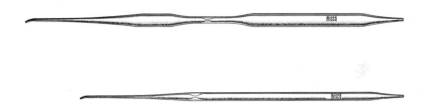

Fig. 5.—Constriction type ultramicro pipets. *Above:* Lang-Levy pipet. *Below:* Lang-Levy type modified for clinical laboratory use.

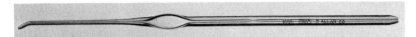

Fig. 6.—KMP constriction type pipet, designed by authors for clinical laboratory use.

type of pipet are given by Natelson.[4] In his pipet the site of construction is the end of a little cylinder enclosed within the lumen. Construction of polyethylene constriction pipets is described by Mattenheimer.[4a, 4b]

The authors have used the constriction-type pipet almost exclusively for routine hospital ultramicro analytical work. It has the advantages of accuracy, simplicity of design, and ease of cleaning. It is considerably less complicated to manufacture than most of the overflow varieties and does not require the use of the squeeze bottle or the syringe type pipet control needed for straight pipets. In the course of developing ultramicro methods and equipment, the advisability of incorporating several modifications into the Lang-Levy constriction pipet became apparent (Fig. 5). With the help of a laboratory equipment company, a constriction-type pipet* was designed specifically for clinical laboratory use[5] (Fig. 6).

These pipets can be bought precalibrated in sizes of 5 to 500 microliters or "lambdas." The limit of acceptable error has been set at 0.5 per cent for pipets up to 40 microliters in size and plus or minus 0.1 per cent for 50 microliters and larger sizes. The following improvements have been made:

1. All pipets are made to exact size; no calculations are necessary owing to the pipet being slightly larger or smaller than the size required.

2. Pipets are sturdy and built to stand up under use in the clinical laboratory. Breakage has been minimal.

3. They are rapid to use. The constriction is so designed as to permit passage of viscous liquids such as concentrated sulfuric acid. It is considerably easier to handle volatile reagents than with most overflow types.

4. The pipets are long enough so that the tip will extend to the bottom of a 7 × 70 mm. test tube (a type commonly used in ultramicro laboratories) or

---

* "KMP" Lang-Levy type pipets, Richard-Allan Co., Inc.

will enter ultramicro blood collection tubes. The tip is beveled and curved slightly.

5. There is no calibration line. Fluid automatically stops at the constriction when the pipet is tilted.

Overflow Pipets

The overflow pipet can be designed to produce the greatest precision. with commercially available pycnometer types measuring as little as 0.1 lambdas. Methods for their construction have been described by Natelson[4] and Murayama.[6] Because these pipets are expensive, difficult to clean, and tend to be wasteful of serum, the constriction pipet has been more widely used in hospital laboratories in the United States. As a result of the work of Sanz,[7-10] as introduced in the United States by Beckman/Spinco, plastic or glass pipets of overflow type have now become very popular (Figs. 7 and 8). The overflow pipets are usually employed as either sample or reagent pipets in conjunction with a small plastic squeeze bottle. An orifice in the plastic or glass dome of the bottle permits delicate finger-tip control over the pipet. Both the Spinco and Coleman systems provide optional aspirator tubes to use in place of the plastic squeeze bottles when pipetting samples, and some technologists find they can control samples better in this way.

Plastic pipets have the advantage that they are flexible (and thus less susceptible to breakage) and provide non-wettable surfaces. Reliability varies in proportion to the degree of quality control over the manufacturing process; drawn pipets seem more accurate than the molded ones. Glass pipets may be silicone-coated; their fragile tips should be carefully protected. Color-coding of the polyethylene plugs holding the pipets, as introduced by Coleman, should prove valuable as indicators of the sizes, as pipets of this caliber are difficult to label clearly or with permanence (Fig. 9).

A reagent pipet has a plastic tube extending nearly to the base of the bottle through which reagent reaches the dome containing the inner end of the pipet. In order to prevent the reagent from squirting out of the orifice at the top, Spinco bottles are now fitted with plastic "bugs" and Coleman's with plastic bands which divert the reagent stream (Fig. 10).

Calibration of Pipets

The calibration of pipets may be checked with mercury, drawing it up to the point of constriction or overflow and weighing the expelled contents.[11] Other methods of calibration use water or methylene iodide;[12] colorimetric methods use phenosulfonphthalein,[4] chromic sulfate,[13, 14] or titrate 0.1 N NaCl standard vs. 0.005 N mercuric nitrate.[4]

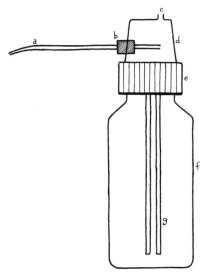

Fig. 7.—Schematic drawing of an overflow pipet. The pipet (a) is of drawn plastic or glass, held in place by a color-coded plug (b) inserted in the plastic dome (d). The pipet is controlled by means of the plastic squeeze bottle (f) and an orifice (c) in the dome. Reagent pipets are equipped with a tube (g) extending close to the bottom of the reservoir; sample pipets are similar, but without the tube (g).

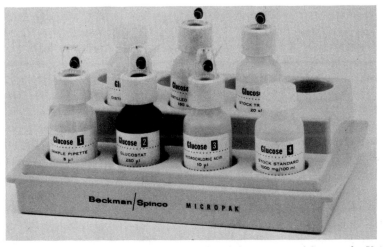

Fig. 8.—Beckman/Spinco ultramicro pipets introduced the concepts of Sanz to the United States. Clearly-labeled plastic squeeze bottles are numbered in the order of their use in a procedure. The pipets are designed either for measurement of the sample or the reagents; they are of drawn plastic and of overflow type.

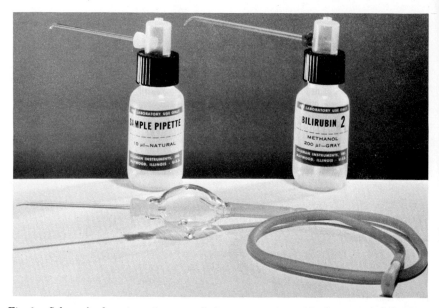

Fig. 9.—Coleman's ultramicro pipets are of glass construction, with plastic squeeze bottles. Note color coding of plugs holding the overflow pipets in the plastic domes. The system also provides an all-glass detachable pipet for sampling (foreground).

To calibrate constriction-type pipets to contain, weigh the pipet and then draw in mercury to the point of constriction. The mercury and the pipet are then weighed together and the weight of the pipet is subtracted from the total. The weight of the mercury divided by 13.5461 (specific gravity of mercury) equals the volume of the pipet. Temperature differences between 20 C. and 30 C. affect the mercury column only about one-tenth of a lambda (0.0001 ml.) and do not need to be considered for our purposes. Volume of a pipet calibrated to contain may be reduced by filing down the tip of the pipet and then re-weighing with mercury.

In the colorimetric method described by Ellerbrook[14, 15] a moderately colored "standard" solution is prepared by measuring out a known volume of a stable, strongly colored stock solution with an accurate volumetric pipet and adding it to a measured volume of diluent (at least 10 and preferably 100 volumes). The same stock solution measured from the pipet to be calibrated is added to exactly the same proportion of diluent. The two diluted colored solutions are read in the same photometer tube. The size of the tubes and the wavelength of the light are adjusted to give optical densities of 0.3 to 0.5, near the region of least instrumental error. The volume delivered by

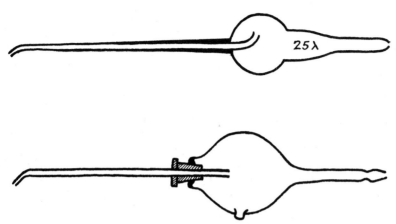

Fig. 10.—Schematic drawing of glass overflow pipets. *Above:* A fine glass tube of uniform bore empties into a waste chamber. *Below:* Coleman overflow pipets can be detached from the plastic squeeze bottles and inserted in a waste chamber, or "pig," controlled by an aspirator tube. The size of the pipet is indicated by the color-coded plastic plug.

the pipet being calibrated is calculated from the ratio of the optical densities of the "standard" and "unknown" colored solutions.

The reliability of the results may be increased by using the average reading of several standards prepared with different containers and by making replicate pipettings with the pipets to be calibrated. The accuracy of the method increases with the dilution of the stock colored solution, as long as reasonable final optical densities are maintained. Potassium dichromate solutions are convenient colored solutions to use. Two ml. of a 1 per cent aqueous solution of potassium dichromate added to 100 ml. of water and read in a 19 mm. cuvet for the Coleman Junior Spectrophotometer gives optical densities of about 0.500, 0.350, and 0.125 at wavelengths of 400, 450, and 500 mμ, respectively.

A method using an aqueous concentration of nicotinamide is described by Dixit and Lazarow.[15a] The absorbence is read in a spectrophotometer at 262 mμ, and the volume of the micropipet is calculated by comparing the extinction with that obtained using macro dilutions.

Use of Pipets

Constriction Type: Samples of serum are removed from the capillary tube by the desired size of constriction pipet. Rubber aspirator tubes and glass or plastic mouthpieces are attached to these pipets to facilitate their use. The pipets should first be rinsed with the serum to be tested and this sample then discarded. Serum is drawn to a point just past the constriction and the suction is stopped while the tip of the pipet still remains below the surface. The serum retreats to the point of constriction and is now ready to be transferred, but one must be careful that none adheres to the external surface of the pipet. Proper care can help to avoid hemolysis and the resulting falsely high potassium and phosphate levels.

Overflow Type: No less care is required for use of overflow pipets. The elaborate directions for the use of the Spinco and Coleman varieties are presented in their instruction manuals, so it would be superfluous to go into details here. The following suggestions may be found useful:

1. When first learning to use overflow pipets, be particularly careful in pipetting samples, as it is easy to lose the sample.

2. Practice pipetting more volatile reagents, such as alcohol, before assuming you have mastered the technic.

3. Check the tops of the plastic squeeze bottles to see that the rims are perfectly round and smooth. This is important to prevent leakage of air during the pipetting process.

4. If possible, always use the same bottle for sampling, interchanging the pipets. This enables you to become accustomed to the amount of pressure used and to achieve more precise control.

5. Always use the same pipet for measuring the standard and unknown. This principle holds for all types of pipets and minimizes possible errors in calibration.

6. Beware of bubbles entrapped within the pipet. Also, be sure no drops of liquid remain adherent to the inside wall after the pipet has been emptied.

Straight Type: The straight capillary pipets are very precise when used with syringe type pipet controls. They have received extensive use in dealing with radioactive isotopes, but they require two hands to manipulate and adoption for ultramicro procedures in clinical laboratories has been quite limited. They are particularly useful in achieving greater degrees of accuracy in pipetting liquid in amount of 50 microliters or less, where the constriction type pipet is less reliable. Wilkinson[16] describes their use in clinical medicine in England. Reagent type pipets are calibrated to deliver; sample pipets are calibrated to contain. He emphasizes the importance of training the technician in the proper "washing out" technic to deliver serum or plasma to 1 per cent accuracy.

Care of Pipets

Contamination is such a serious problem in ultramicro chemistry, and the quantities pipetted are so minute, that pipets must be kept scrupulously clean.

As with any pipet, prompt cleaning after each use will minimize cleaning problems. If bubbles form within the pipet or drops remain on the surface, the pipet needs cleaning. Glass constriction-type pipets may be filled with detergent, concentrated nitric acid, or potassium dichromate solution, allowed to stand for several hours, then rinsed at least 20 times with distilled water. Contamination may be reduced by reserving specific pipets for each method.

The Spinco manual recommends removal of the invisible film of protein within the plastic sample pipets by filling each evening with a fresh solution of 0.1 N HCl containing 0.5 per cent pepsin. By morning, the digestive action of pepsin will have removed this film. The use of ammonium hydroxide for cleaning the reagent pipets should be avoided in any analyses involving the production of ammonia. *Never* use a stylet on a plastic pipet. An ultrasonic cleaner is sometimes successful in removing firm particles from within the lumen of a pipet or micro test tube.

Sources of Pipets

Coleman Instruments, Inc., Maywood, Ill.
Kimble Glass Co., Toledo 1, Ohio
Microchemical Specialties Co., 1825 Eastshore Hwy., Berkeley 10, Calif.
Research Specialties Co., 200 South Garrard Blvd., Richmond, Calif.
Richard-Allan Co., 1335 Dodge Ave., Evanston, Ill.
Scientific Products, Div., American Hospital Supply Co., Evanston, Ill.
Spinco Div., Beckman Instrument Corp., 1117 California Ave., Palo Alto, Calif.

BURETS

Ultramicro burets are not only considerably more accurate than their larger counterparts, they are generally easier to use. They are available in two varieties—those employing a plunger of uniform diameter to displace a measured volume of fluid, and those in which the liquid is forced out by a plunger immersed in mercury. In the latter, the surface of the advancing column of mercury acts as an indicator against the calibrated wall of the glass tubing, or a micrometer may record the advance of the plunger.

Many modifications of each type are available, including semi-automatic and automatic burets (Fig. 11), and featuring such refinements as mechanical stirring attachments. In the hospital laboratory the calibrated plunger type has proved both sturdy and reliable, and as the presence of mercury may contaminate the reagent,[18] an instrument such as the Gilmont[19] micropipet-buret*

---

* Available from the Manostat Corp., New York 13, N. Y.

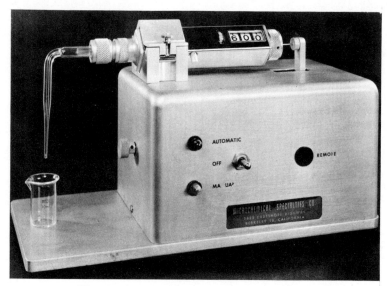

Fig. 11.—Automatic buret with a digital counter.

can be recommended (Fig. 12). It should be kept in mind that if more than one substance (e.g., chloride and calcium) is to be measured by titrimetric procedures, two burets will be needed to provide efficient service.

Gilmont Micropipet-Buret

The Gilmont micropipet-buret used should have a capacity of 1.0 ml. in 0.001 ml. divisions. Originally manufactured with a dial gauge, recent models are provided with a digital counter reading to three places. The titrating fluid comes in contact only with the glass plunger and the tetrafluorethylene gasket. To fill the instrument, the plunger is extended to its maximum and solution is sucked back into the reservoir by retracting the plunger about three-quarters of the way. Remove the buret from the liquid, retract the plunger fully, tilt the tip of the instrument up and tap the chamber lightly until all air is at the capillary end. Force out the air bubble by advancing the plunger, then continue with the filling process. It is sometimes necessary to repeat this procedure one or more times until the instrument is completely filled. To check for the presence of air entrapped in the instrument, observe the meniscus near the end of the glass tip, with the tip first held up, then down. Movement of the meniscus as a result of inverting the instrument is an indication of entrapped air.

The micropipet-buret is mounted on a laboratory stand by means of a double

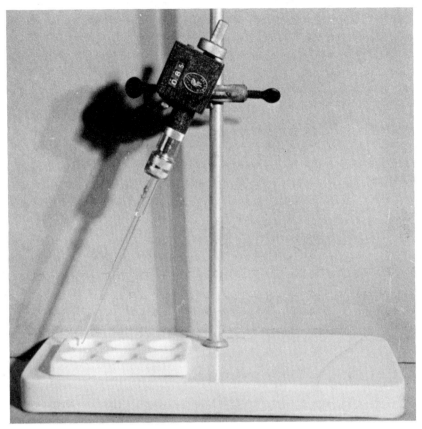

Fig. 12.—Gilmont micropipet-buret, 1.0 ml. capacity.

clamp. Titration is best done into a spot plate using a glass rod for stirring. The buret tip is kept just below the liquid surface to avoid the effect of surface tension or the error of a hanging drop.

Spinco Microtitrator and Coleman Microtrator

The Spinco Microtitrator* (Fig. 13) and the Coleman Microtrator† (Fig. 14) are both micrometer-driven and horizontally mounted. Their comparative features are presented here:

---

* Beckman/Spinco Co., Palo Alto, Calif.
† Coleman Instruments, Inc., Maywood, Ill.

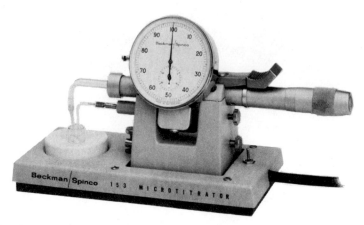

Fig. 13.—Beckman/Spinco Microtitrator. The plunger (not visible) is advanced by turning the knurled handle, expelling fluid through the plastic buret tip into the titrating cup. Mixing is done by means of a vibrating plastic tip extending below the surface level. Positioning of the buret and vibrating tip may be accurately controlled.

	Spinco Microtitrator	*Coleman Microtrator*
Capacity	500 microliters	190 microliters
Indicator device	Dial gauge	Digital readout counter
Reset mechanism	Zero button	Counter reset disc
Mixing	Adjustable vibrating stirrer	Rotating sample cup
Buret tip	Plastic	Plastic
Sample containers	Clear plastic cup	Clear plastic cup
Cup rack capacity	21	24

The Spinco instrument is of somewhat heavier construction and is readily adaptable for the use of a Conway cell or a multiple titrating platform. Its adjustable vibrating tip provides better mixing. The Coleman Microtrator mixes by means of the buret tip suspended over the rotating sample container, and there is a tendency toward layering of liquids of different specific gravity. In both instruments the heights of the buret tips are adjustable. The disposable clear plastic sample containers are well designed and reduce the possibilities of contamination. Neither buret is especially simple to fill, but the Coleman detaches from its base with greater ease. Both reservoirs, and particularly the

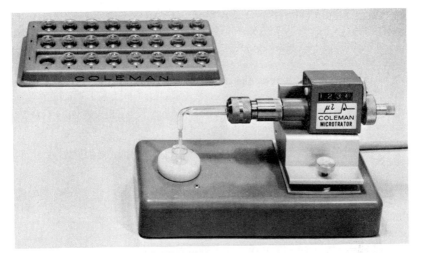

Fig. 14.—Coleman Microtrator. The buret is on a hinged base; dropping it into position activates the rotating platform holding the titration cup. The digital counter measures the reagent in microliters.

Coleman, could be improved by providing greater capacity and reducing the frequency that refilling is required.

Ultra-Buret Model 200 and Gilmont Ultramicro Buret

The Ultra-Buret Model 200,* designed by Natelson,[20] is an instrument of the micrometer screw type; the Gilmont Ultramicro Buret† (not to be confused with the micropipet-buret described previously) is somewhat similar in design. Both use mercury between the plungers and the reagents.

	Ultra-Buret Model 200	Gilmont Ultramicro Buret
Capacity	50 ml. reservoir; 7 ml. without refilling	1.0, 0.1, and 0.01 ml.
Markings	0.001 ml.	1.0 ml. in 0.0001 ml. 0.1 ml. in 0.00001 ml. 0.01 ml. in 0.000001 ml.
Reset	Turn index	Use zero adjusting screw
Mixing	No provision	Bubble tube and support optional equipment
Height	Adjustable	Not adjustable

* Scientific Industries, Springfield, Mass.
† Manostat Corp., New York 13, N. Y.

The Ultra-Buret's chief advantage is its broad range and its large fluid reservoir. The Gilmont is available in three sizes; convenient attachments are available so that mixing may be accomplished by means of bubbles from an air source. Its fixed height is sometimes a disadvantage. The Gilmont counter is rather cumbersome to return to the zero point, but is probably still more satisfactory than reading the micrometer scale. Greatly improved sample mixing can be provided by the use of magnetic devices. Construction of "microflea" stirrers for use with microburets has been described by O'Mara and Faulkner.[47]

Burets of Other Types

Many other burets have been designed, and a number of these are commercially available. Kirk has summarized their earlier development.[12] Some of the modifications of the Rehberg burets are unsuitable for the clinical laboratory—fragile construction, excessive size, high mercury pressure, inadequate capacity, and difficulties in reading are all factors mitigating against their use. Kirk has designed modifications of the Rehberg-type buret and also an improved version of the Schwarz buret.* The latter is horizontally mounted, and automatically maintains a small, constant hydrostatic pressure which is controlled by the finely drawn tip.

A buret which has received some clinical acceptance is that of Lazarow,† which interchanges various sizes of ground glass syringes and buret tips. A dial indicator records the amount of fluid expelled.[13] A microburet attachment is available for the Natelson Microgasometer.‡ One of the authors (E.M.K.) has designed a buret with a vertically mounted plunger and a universal joint at the top to facilitate filling the instrument. Automatic burets are available from the American Instrument Co., Labline, Inc., and Microchemical Specialties, Inc., but these are not required unless there is a very high volume of laboratory work.

Choosing a Buret

Selection of a buret for the clinical laboratory must take into account the factors of cost, reliability, durable construction, ease of repair, and availability of service. The number of burets required for an ultramicro chemical laboratory depends upon how many different titrimetric procedures are to be used. A separate buret is needed for each reagent, as it is most impractical to attempt to clean and refill the reagent reservoirs between procedures.

---

* Microchemical Specialties, Inc., Berkeley, Calif.
† Micrometric Instrument Co., Cleveland, Ohio.
‡ Scientific Industries, Inc., Springfield, Mass.

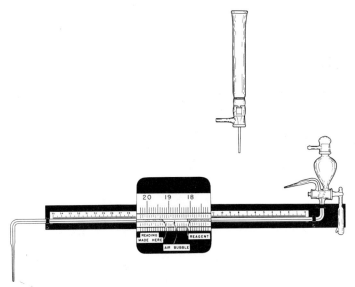

Fig. 15.—Grunbaum-Kirk buret with automatic reagent supply.

The size and design of the tip of the buret is most important to its proper function. The tip is kept just under the surface of the liquid during the titrations, and if the bore is too wide there will be backflow of fluid and some of the reaction will take place inside the tip of the instrument. If the buret has a plastic tip, it should be inspected carefully to assure that there is no leakage at the joint between the glass and plastic. Leakage at the other end, i.e., around the plunger, may be even more serious, as it not only results in inaccuracy but some reagent may seep into mechanical parts and cause corrosion.

Mercury-containing burets, while very accurate, are not essential for hospital laboratory work. The plunger types must be checked, however, to insure that there is uniformity of the caliber of the plunger in all areas. Sanz[7] comments that glass pistons tend to be thinner at their centers than at the ends, and differences in diameter as little as 0.1 to 0.5 per cent may adversely affect titrimetric procedures measured in the microliter range. He recommends the use of metal pistons which are rhodium-plated.

Either the height of the buret or that of the titrating platform should be easily adjustable. Design of the titrating cups is also important; deeper cups minimize the hazards of contamination but require much better illumination to bring out subtle titrimetric end-points. Mechanical mixing, while more spectacular, is sometimes difficult to control and the time-honored stirring rod is entirely satisfactory for nearly all titrations. Directions are available for construction of magnetic mixing devices.[47]

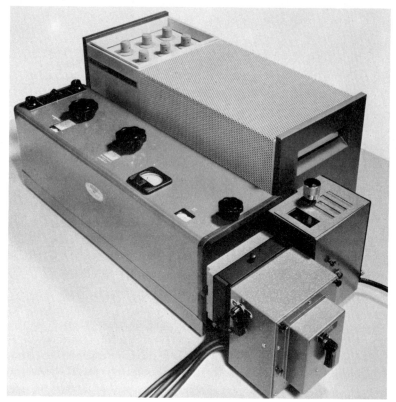

Fig. 16.—Beckman DU Spectrophotometer.

SPECTROPHOTOMETERS

Beckman DU Spectrophotometer

The Beckman DU spectrophotomoter (Fig. 16) has been modified for ultra-micro analysis[22, 23] and is particularly suitable because of its narrow beam of monochromatic light and sensitive photometer for light detection. For the clinical laboratory, the Bessey-Lowry cells recommended by Caraway[24] are easy to manipulate. (Pyrocell Mfg. Co.; Quaracell Products, Inc.) They are of fused silica, which is highly transparent over the entire spectral range of the DU. They have an inside chamber measuring 2.5 × 10 × 25 mm. and are used with a cell carrier and diaphragm attachment. An adapter is available which permits the use of the Craig rotary cell holder.[25] (Microchemical Specialties Co.)

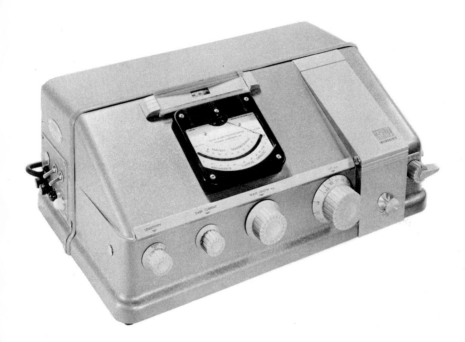

Fig. 17.—Beckman B Spectrophotometer.

An alternative approach is the use of capillary cells, of which two types are available. In the small bore type, the ends are covered by cover slips held in place by capillary action. The larger caliber tubes have clip-on ends holding the windows in place. The advantage of the capillary cells is that they provide a longer light absorption path for a given volume of solution, thus permitting greater accuracy.[26] A disadvantage is the increased difficulty in filling, which has been partially overcome by Sobel.[27]

Beckman B Spectrophotometer

The Beckman B spectrophotometer (Fig. 17) can be adapted to ultramicro work using either the Bessey-Lowry cells or capillary cells. The width of the light beam is already controllable and height may be easily reduced by the use of opaque electrician's tape on the masking plate. The instrument is not capable of the precision of the DU model; however, we have used the Model B on a standby basis.

SPECTROPHOTOMETER CHARACTERISTICS

Features	Beckman DU	Beckman/Spinco Colorimeter	Coleman Jr. Ultramicro Assembly
Light source	Hydrogen discharge tube (210-400 mμ), tungsten bulb (330-1000 mμ)	Tungsten lamp	Tungsten lamp, 6V
Dispersion	Quartz prism	Glass wedge interference filter; auxiliary filters	Diffraction grating
Slit widths	to 1 mμ	15 mμ	35 mμ
Range	210-1000 mμ	400-650 mμ	350-700 mμ
Cuvet emptying	Manual	Vacuum pump	Vacuum pump
Photo element	Phototubes with amplifier	Phototube and amplifier	Barrier layer photocell
Ultramicro cuvet*	Quartz, 10 mm. light path	Glass, 6.4 mm. light path	Glass, 10 mm. light path

* Subject to change or substitution.

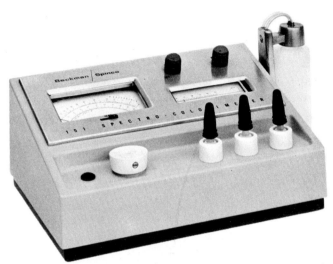

Fig. 18.—Beckman/Spinco Model 151 Spectro-Colorimeter. This instrument has a flow-through cuvet for ultramicro analysis; micro and macro cuvets may also be used. A suction pump drains the cuvet contents into a waste bottle.

Beckman/Spinco Colorimeter

The Beckman/Spinco Model 151 Spectro-Colorimeter is the first such instrument to be introduced primarily for clinical ultramicro chemical analysis (although other larger cuvets are available) and is a direct-reading combination photoelectric spectrophotometer and colorimeter. This instrument considerably lowers the cost of installing ultramicro methods and is one of the most significant contributions to the field in recent years (Fig. 18).

The Model 151 provides wave lengths over a range of 400 to 650 mμ with the glass wedge interference filter, with a band width of approximately 15 mμ. Auxiliary filters may be used. The light source is a fixed-focus low wattage tungsten lamp. The cuvet is of flow-through type, emptying into a waste bottle by means of a vacuum pump. The photoelectric current is indicated by a meter in both absorbance and per cent transmittance. Three dropper type wash bottles are built into the instrument; these normally contain distilled water, a detergent solution, and 1 per cent caprylic alcohol in acetone.

Coleman Junior Ultramicro Cell Assembly

The Coleman Junior Spectrophotometer can be adapted for ultramicro quantities by means of an ultramicro cell assembly. This is comprised of an ultramicro cell adapter and cell, wash rack and wash bottles, transfer pipets, and

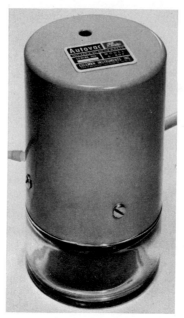

Fig. 19.—Autovac pump for emptying Coleman ultramicro cuvets.

the Coleman Autovac Pump with tubing and reservoir (Fig. 19). The ultra-micro cell (#6-803) (Fig. 20) is rectangular, with a volume of 100 micro-liters and a light path of 1.0 cm. The adapter (Fig. 21) holds and positions an aspirating tube, which, when depressed, exhausts the cell's contents into the separate Autovac Pump reservoir via a drain tube.

The band width of the Model 6A or Model 6C Junior Spectrophotometer is approximately 35 mμ. The range is from 400 to 700 mμ.

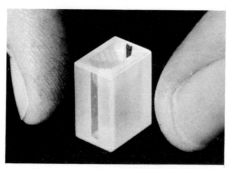

Fig. 20.—Coleman's ultramicro cell, featuring a 1 cm. light path.

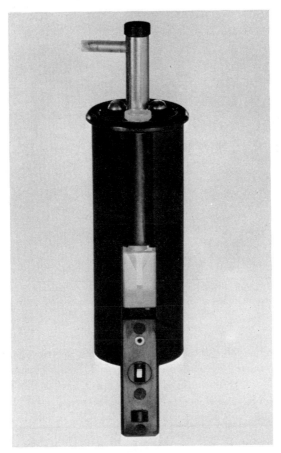

Fig. 21.—Coleman ultramicro cell adapter permits ultramicro analysis in the Coleman Junior Spectrophotometer. An aspirator assembly may be depressed to empty the cuvet by suction.

Other Instruments

Other instruments which have been used for ultramicro methods include the Evelyn colorimeter with microcell attachment, the Evans single cell photoelectric absorptiometer and the Spekker two cell photoelectric absorptiometer.[16] A micro space adapter and one-half inch round cuvet for the Bausch and Lomb Spectronic 20 Colorimeter measures volumes as small as 1 ml. Sanz has used the Beckman C colorimeter with a specially designet cuvet.[7] A good discussion of submicrogram analysis equipment is given by Kirk in his *Quan-*

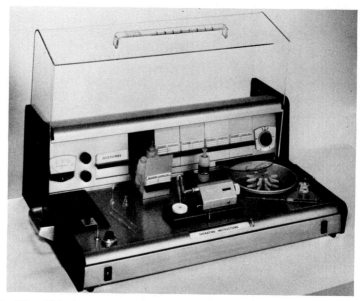

Fig. 22.—Misco Teknikit, a semi-portable unit with built-in photometer, hot plate, buret, centrifuge, and reagent drawers. Operating instructions are on a centrally located roller. (Microchemical Specialties Co.)

titative Ultramicroanalysis.[12] The section on colorimetric analysis in Milton and Waters' *Methods of Quantitative Analysis* is also recommended.[28]

A recent addition to the ultramicro equipment field is the Teknikit manufactured by Microchemical Specialties Co. Measuring only 12″ high by 25″ deep by 36″ wide, this semi-portable unit includes a micro photometer, an electric heating block, a microburet and a microcentrifuge. Reagent drawers are built into the back of the unit. Another feature is a built-in fluorescent lamp which turns on when the clear plexiglas cover is tilted back. Polyethylene reagent bottles are provided for reagents; some of these have pipetting systems operated by the simple depression of a plunger. 110 V AC operates the unit (Fig. 22).

FLAME PHOTOMETERS

Measurement of serum sodium and potassium is accomplished on the ultramicro scale by means of emission spectrophotometry. The large number of clinical flame photometers available commercially permits the pathologist or biochemist to select a model most adaptable to his own laboratory. He may wish to have a flame photometer combined with a spectrophotometer, or he may prefer to have a separate instrument set aside for the specific use of the ultramicro division of his laboratory.

Basically all flame photometers are composed of an atomizer, a burner assembly with flame, an optical system, one or more photoelectric cells, and a galvanometer. Flame photometers are available in two types: the single photocell instrument and the double photocell, or "internal standard" variety.

In *single photocell* types, the relative intensity of spectroemission of a substance is measured in terms of per cent transmission or net luminosity as compared with one or more standards measured under identical conditions. Variations in air, oxygen or gas pressure, rate of aspiration of the sample, or optical system changes will cause errors in the determination. The presence of interfering substances either in the solution being measured or in the gases will also cause erroneous results unless the substances are present in approximately the same concentration in the standards as in the unknowns. An advantage of this type of photometer is that it may be used for calcium measurements.

The *double photocell* (internal standard) type of flame photometer utilizes balanced photocells. One photocell is activated by an internal standard added to the sample in known quantities; lithium is the element most commonly used in the clinical laboratory. The output of the phototube activated by the lithium standard is balanced against the output of the other phototube activated by the unknown sample under identical conditions. This approach effectively eliminates the sources of error found in the single photocell type of flame photometer, although variations in concentration of other interfering ions in serum and variations in flame temperature may introduce other errors into the analysis.

Numerous excellent flame photometers are available.[20, 39] The only criterion for their adaptation to ultramicro use is that they be sufficiently sensitive to permit the use of a fairly high dilution of the small amounts of serum available. The chapter on Sodium and Potassium discusses the use of the Advanced, Baird, and Coleman instruments. The Advanced and Baird are reliable flame photometers using an internal lithium standard. The Advanced's chief advantages are its small size (8½" x 7"), simplicity of construction, and relatively low price (Fig. 23). The Baird Model KY-1 has combined the accuracy of the internal standard method with the ease of reading of the single photocell, direct reflection instruments (Fig. 24). Both are well shielded from airborne contamination. The Coleman is of the single beam, direct reading type and may be used with a Coleman Junior spectrophotometer or Galvo-O-Meter. A microcell is available, and the instrument may also be used for calcium determinations (Fig. 25).

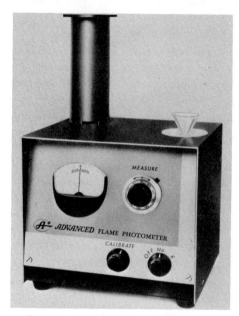

Fig. 23.—Advanced Flame Photometer.

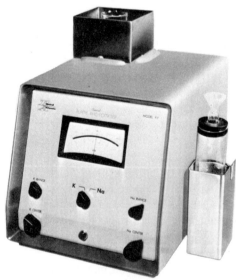

Fig. 24.—Baird-Atomic Flame Photometer, Model KY.

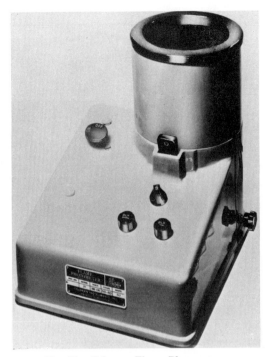

Fig. 25.—Coleman Flame Photometer.

CENTRIFUGES

Several types of centrifuges have been used in conjunction with clinical ultramicro analysis. They are used for three specific purposes:

1) Separation of plasma or serum from the blood cells.

2) Separation of precipitate from supernatant fluid during chemical analysis. This method is used almost exclusively in preference to filtration.

3) Performance of microhematocrits. Although not a part of ultramicro analysis, the micro-hematocrit test frequently accompanies the chemical procedures. See the chapter on Microhematocrits for a detailed description of centrifuges available.

A standard model of any reliable centrifuge is satisfactory for centrifugation of clotted blood collected in capillary tubes since the capped or sealed tubes may be placed within macro-sized tubes for spinning.

For separation in the 1.0 ml. ultramicro centrifuge tubes, a Misco (Microchemical Specialties Co.) electric microcentrifuge may be used. This is a sturdily-built model modified from Kirk's air turbine ultramicro centrifuge[30]

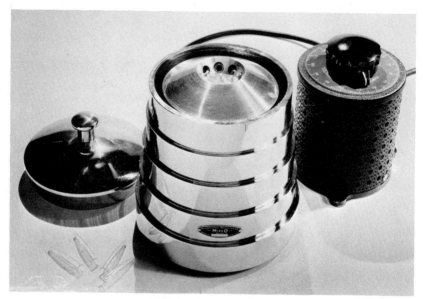

Fig. 26.—Misco Ultramicro Centrifuge with rheostat.

and provides speeds up to 22,000 rpm controlled by a separate rheostat (Fig. 26). The centrifuge holds eight narrow-lipped tubes. Another micro-chemistry centrifuge is manufactured by Clay-Adams. Holding eight tubes, this centrifuge has a maximum speed of 13,500 rpm. An electric brake stops the head in 60 seconds, and there is a built-in timer. The International Model MB may be used with an eight-place head at 15,000 rpm. The International clinical centrifuge with an angle head gives somewhat lower speeds.

The Beckman/Spinco Microfuge (Fig. 27) is a cleverly-designed instrument providing rapid acceleration and deceleration. Instead of a head it has a rotator with four vertical slots in the rotator walls. Metal slides, each with five punched holes for five tubes, fit into the vertical slots. The tubes are of polyethylene construction, with caps, and are held in place by the flared lips. They hold 400 microliters and are discarded after use. Tube racks are provided with numbered holes matching numbers on the vertical slides.

The Coleman centrifuge also has a rotor containing four vertical tube holders. It provides rapid acceleration and is said to exceed 13,000 rpm and 10,800 g in 4 seconds with a full load. It spins capped polyethylene tubes of 400 microliter capacity; identification is preserved by lettering on the tube holders and the tube rack (Fig. 28).

The rotor ultramicro centrifuge, as introduced by Spinco, seems to represent a significant advance in centrifugation technic. The Spinco centrifuge

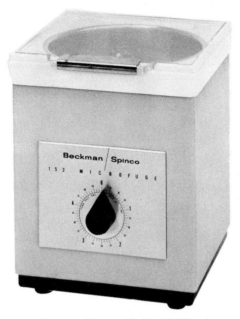

Fig. 27.—Beckman/Spinco Model 152 Microfuge.

is slightly smaller in overall size than the Coleman. Both are quite noisy in operation, but this is also true of the Misco centrifuge.

Microgasometer

The Natelson microgasometer (Model 600, Scientific Industries, Inc.) is used for gas content analyses.[4, 20, 31, 32] It is a manometric instrument based on the classic Van Slyke method. The mercury reservoir is controlled by a hand wheel and gas pressure is measured under constant volume so that results are not dependent on atmospheric pressure. Serum samples of only 0.03 ml. are required. Complete instructions for the use of this instrument are supplied by the manufacturer.

Accessories available for the microgasometer include a microburet attachment and a motorized shaker attachment. The latter is useful if large numbers of tests are performed; it is provided with a timer for periods up to 5 minutes. An optional background lighting device provides uniform lighting of variable intensity and makes the readings considerably easier (Fig. 29). O'Mara and Faulkner describe how to construct a completely mechanized version of the Natelson microgasometer.[48]

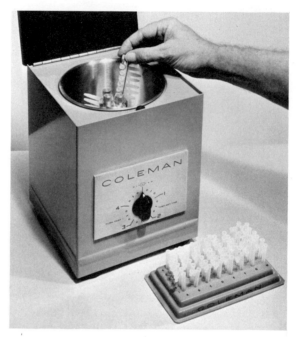

Fig. 28.—Coleman Centrifuge.

pH Meters and Microelectrodes

Rapid progress has been made in the development of pH meters for clinical use since the publication of our first edition. The chapter on Blood pH Measurement describes the use of the Metrohm precision compensator E322 (Brinkmann Instruments, Inc.) with the capillary electrode chain EA 518 designed by Sanz (Fig. 30). An improved version of this instrument is the model E388, reading directly to 0.001 pH; all values are read in a single window. This is used in combination with the pistol grip micro capillary electrode chain (EA 521) and the Haake FSB constant temperature circulator (Fig. 31). Other superior instruments are the pH meter 4 (Fig. 32) and the pH meter 22 made by Radiometer (The London Company). In the Metrohm instrument, the electrode potential is compensated by a calibrated compensating voltage; a cathode ray tube used as the zero indicator eliminates bearing friction. All of these instruments provide for temperature compensation, an essential feature if precision is to be attained. The Radiometer pH meter 4 is a battery-operated instrument providing extremely high accuracy;[33] the pH meter 22 is a direct-reading instrument operating on AC and designed for general laboratory use.

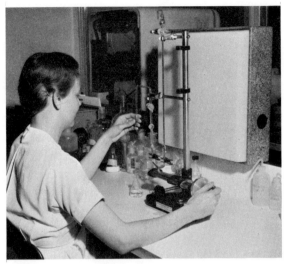

Fig. 29.—Natelson Microgasometer, Model 600 (Scientific Industries, Inc.).

The Beckman model 76 expanded scale pH meter and the Coleman Com-panION pH meter are also available with a variety of electrodes.

The National Bureau of Standards pH standard[44] is designed to facilitate pH measurements in the pH 7-8 range; the buffer solution is composed of KH_2PO_4 and Na_2HPO_4, catalog numbers 186Ib and 186IIb. Determination of blood pCO_2 is discussed extensively by Gambino; he concludes that the most accurate and precise method of determination is with the Severinghaus modi-fication of the pCO_2 electrode.[45, 46]

The accompanying table gives the relative features of two of the better pH meters.

TABLE 2.—pH METERS—COMPARATIVE FEATURES*

	Radiometer pH-Meter 4	Metrohm Model E388
Measuring range	0-14 pH	0-14 pH
Accuracy	.001 pH	0.001 pH
Temperature compensation	Provided	Provided
Circuit	Compensated type	Compensated type
Power	Battery-operated	110, 125, 145, 220, 250 V.

* Supplied by manufacturers.

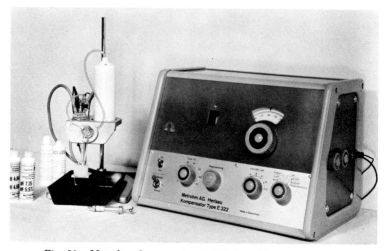

Fig. 30.—Metrohm Compensator E 322 for pH measurement.

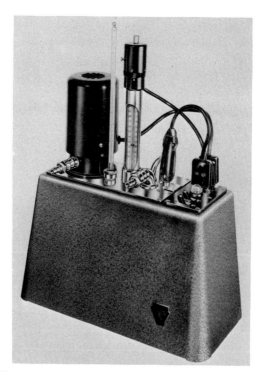

Fig. 31.—Thermostat, Type F, Haake, used with Metrohm pH apparatus.

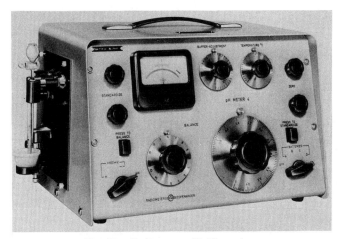

Fig. 32.—Radiometer pH Meter 4.

Another excellent way of measuring pH at the bedside is with the AME1 Astrup micro equipment, but this requires a substantially greater investment. In order to determine the pCO_2, standard bicarbonate, base excess and buffer base, two blood samples, stabilized with heparin are transferred to two small thermostatted and vibrated glass tubes. They are equilibrated with humidified CO_2-O_2 mixtures of known carbon dioxide tensions, then drawn into the glass electrode and the pH is measured. In a nomogram with the pH as the abscissa and the log pCO_2 as the ordinate, the relation between pH and log pCO_2 will be a straight line. This line is determined by the two measured pH values of the equilibrated blood and the corresponding CO_2 tensions. The pCO_2, standard bicarbonate, excess base and buffer base can be read from this nomogram.

An instrument for micro pH determinations has also been designed by Natelson (Scientific Industries, Inc.).

PAPER ELECTROPHORESIS EQUIPMENT

For the performance of paper electrophoresis in the clinical laboratory there is a wide choice of commercially available equipment, or one may choose to construct one's own equipment following one of the many examples given in the literature.[34-42] Two systems described here represent combinations which have proven satisfactory, but there is no intention to imply superiority over other apparatus.

LKB 3276BN Paper Electrophoresis Apparatus

This apparatus is selected because of simplicity of design, reproducibility of results as compared with Tiselius equipment, reliability and moderate cost. The LKB paper electrophoresis apparatus is supplied in the United States by Ivan Sorval, Inc. It is designed for use with the LKB 3290B power supply, connecting to 11, 127, 220, or 240 volts AC and provides a maximum output of 50 milliamperes at 275 volts with milliampere ranges of 0-10 and 0-50   A voltmeter is included in the power supply. The 3276BN instrument provides for horizontal orientation of four 40 mm. wide filter strips or a 2.5 mm. maximum thickness starch gel layer, and it has a protecting cassette constructed with three transverse slits to allow a choice of starting points. A safety switch which disconnects the power supply when the lid is opened is another desirable feature. A sample applicator is available (LKB 3276-SA).

A semiautomatic densitometer (Photovolt Densitometer Model 425, Photovolt Corp.) may be used with this instrument to evaluate the paper strips. A completely automatic recording densitometer is to be desired where the factors of time and volume play an important role, but this semiautomatic instrument is vastly superior to the time-consuming and tedious process of elution. The optical transmission densities are measured by a barrier-layer type self generating photocell sealed into transparent plastic. The machine is used with a guide that will accommodate paper strips up to 40 mm. wide. Results are recorded in a semiautomatic manner, although an automatic electric recorder is available for use with this instrument. While this densitometer records optical transmission, one using reflected light has also been described.

Spinco Model R Electrophoresis Apparatus

This three-part system is extensively used in this country. It consists of a Durrum-type electrophoresis cell, the Duostat power unit, and the Analytrol. The electrophoresis cell holds eight 12" strips of filter paper in an inverted V arrangement and uses baffled platinum electrodes. The fluid level remains balanced. The power unit provides current from 3 to 40 milliamperes or constant voltage of 80 to 500 volts. Two electrophoresis cell units may be operated from the power supply. The Analytrol automatically scans the paper electrophoresis strips and converts the color density pattern into a concentration curve. A second pen draws a series of "pips," summing up the total area under the peaks. A micro-applicator is also available.

OTHER EQUIPMENT

Some other items of equipment will be needed for completely outfitting the ultramicro laboratory. These are listed below:

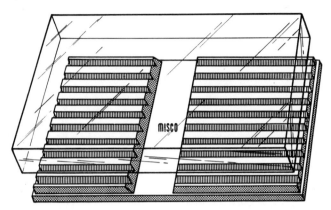

Fig. 33.—Misco ultramicro pipet rack with clear plastic cover.

Micro electric hotplate: The micro electric hotplate recommended by Caraway[24] (#6169L, A. H. Thomas Co.; Thermolyne 42-711, Eberbach & Son) and fitted with a stainless steel, spun aluminum, or copper bowl is ideal for ultramicro use. A circular test tube rack can then be constructed of aluminum or copper to fit the bowl.

Water bath: Many satisfactory serologic water baths are available commercially. A constant level water bath may be used with the micro electric hotplate (83865, Aloe).

Pipet racks: These are necessary to protect the constriction or straight pipets from breakage. Constructed of wood or plastic, they are provided with clear plastic covers (Microchemical Specialties Co.) (Figs. 33 and 34).

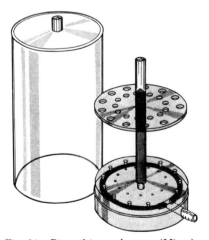

Fig. 34.—Pipet drier and cover (Misco).

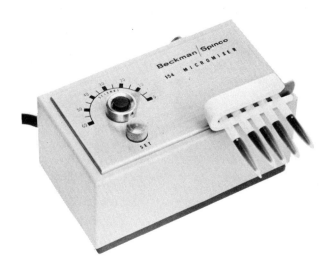

Fig. 35.—Beckman/Spinco Micromixer.

Spot plates: These may be either of the glazed porcelain variety or of clear Pyrex to permit the use of various colored backgrounds for contrast. The wells are used for titration with the Gilmont micropipet-buret.

Mixer: Adequate mixing is essential and is rather difficult to achieve in the small centrifuge tubes. Use of a mixer (Spinco mixer (Fig. 35); Vortex Jr. Mixer, Scientific Industries, Inc.) insures complete mixing in the translucent plastic tubes where a good visual check is not possible.

Ultrasonic cleaner: Small pieces of glass equipment and some pipets can be freed of encrusted material by means of ultrasonic waves. The Sonblaster Series 200 (Narda Ultrasonics Corp.) or a similar small ultrasonic cleaner is satisfactory for this purpose.

Additional items include glass-stoppered 10 ml. Pyrex flasks, glass-stoppered 125 ml. Pyrex bottles, 100 ml. and 10 ml. volumetric flasks, 1 ml. and 2 ml. breakers, 2 ml. glass-stoppered test tubes, and 1 ml. narrow lip centrifuge tubes. Tapered rubber stoppers and rubber vial stoppers (#68MS orange #3, West Co.) are also needed.

REFERENCES

1. KIRK, P. L., AND CRAIG, R.: *J. Lab. & Clin. Med. 18:* 81, 1932.
2. SISCO, R. W., CUNNINGHAM, B., AND KIRK, P. L.: *J. Biol. Chem. 139:* 1, 1941.
3. KROGH, A.: *Indust. & Eng. Chem. 7:* 130, 1935.
4. NATELSON, S.: *Am. J. Clin. Path. 21:* 1153, 1951.
4a. MATTENHEIMER, H., AND BORNER, K.: *Mikrochem. Acta* 916-921, 1959.
4b. _____: *J. Lab. & Clin. Med. 58:* 499, 1961.

5. KNIGHTS, E. M., JR., MACDONALD, R. P., AND PLOOMPUU, J.: *Am. J. Clin. Path. 30:* 91, 1958.
6. MURAYAMA, H.: *J. Lab. & Clin. Med. 39:* 795, 1952.
7. SANZ, M. C.: *Clin. Chem. 3:* 406, 1957.
8. ————: *J. Physiol. 49:* 372, 1957.
9. ————: *Roentgen v. Laboratoriumspraxis 10:* 381, 1957.
10. ————: *Chimia 13:* 192, 1959.
11. RAPPAPORT, F.: Rapid Microchemical Methods for Blood and CSF Examination.
11. RAPPAPORT, F.: Rapid Microchemical Methods for Blood and CSF Examination. New York, Grune & Stratton, 1949.
12. KIRK, P. L.: Quantitative Ultramicroanalysis. New York, Wiley, 1950.
13. DUNN, F. L.: *J. Lab. & Clin. Med. 19:* 95, 1933.
14. ELLERBROOK, L. D.: *Am. J. Clin. Path. 24:* 868, 1954.
15. ————: Workshop on Microchemistry—Technique Manual. Chicago, *Am. Soc. Clin. Path.,* 1960.
15a. DIXIT, P. K., AND LAZAROW, A.: *J. Lab. & Clin. Med. 58:* 499, 1961.
16. WILKINSON, R. H.: Chemical Micromethods in Clinical Medicine. Springfield, Ill., Charles C Thomas, 1960.
17. WINGO, W. J., AND JOHNSON, W. H.: *Anal. Chem. 28:* 1215, 1956.
18. CARAWAY, W. T.: Personal communication.
19. GILMONT, R.: *Anal. Chem. 20:* 1109, 1948.
20. NATELSON, S.: Microtechniques of Clinical Chemistry for the Routine Laboratory. Springfield, Ill., Charles C Thomas, 1957.
21. LAZAROW, A.: *J. Lab. & Clin. Med. 35:* 310, 1950.
22. LOWRY, O. H., AND BESSEY, O. A.: *J. Biol. Chem. 163:* 633, 1946.
23. KIRK, P. L., ROSENFELS, R. S., AND HANAHAN, D. J.: *Anal. Chem. 19:* 355, 1947.
24. CARAWAY, W. T., AND FANGER, H.: *Am. J. Clin. Path. 25:* 317, 1955.
25. CRAIG, R., BARTEL, A., AND KIRK, P. L.: *Rev. Sci. Inst. 24:* 49, 1953.
26. SOBEL, A. E., AND HANOK, A.: *Mikrochemie 39:* 51, 1952.
27. ————, AND SNOW, S.: *J. Biol. Chem. 171:* 617, 1947.
28. MILTON, R. F., AND WATERS, W. A.: Methods of Quantitative Microanalysis. 2nd Ed. London, Edward Arnold, Ltd., 1955.
29. TELOH, H. A.: Clinical Flame Photometry. Springfield, Ill., Charles C. Thomas, 1959.
30. KIRK, P. L.: *Microchemie 14:* 1, 1933.
31. HOLADAY, D. A., AND VEROSKY, M.: *J. Lab. & Clin. Med. 47:* 634, 1956.
32. NATELSON, S., AND MENNING, C. M.: *Clin. Chem. 1:* 165, 1955.
33. GAMBINO, S. R.: Workshop on Microchemistry—Pre-Workshop Manual. Chicago, *Am Soc. Clin. Path.* 1960.
34. DURRUM, E. L.: *J. Am. Chem. Soc. 72:* 2943, 1950.
35. TURBA, F., AND ENENKEL, H. J.: *Naturwissenschaften 37:* 93, 1950.
36. CREMER, H. D., AND TISELIUS, A.: *Biochem. Ztschr. 320:* 273, 1950.
37. FLYNN, F. V., AND DE MAYO, P.: *Lancet 261* (2): 235, 1951.
38. NOVERRAZ, M.: *J. Suisse Med. 82:* 880, 1952.
39. LEVIN, B., AND OBERHOLZER, V. G.: *Am. J. Clin. Path. 23:* 205, 1953.
40. OSSERMAN, E. F., AND LAWLOR, D. P.: *Am. J. Med. 18:* 462, 1955.
41. LEDERER, M.: Introduction to Paper Electrophoresis and Related Methods. Amsterdam, Elsevier, 1957.
42. SVENSSON, H.: Ciba Foundation Symposium on Paper Electrophoresis, Boston. Little, Brown & Co., 1956, p. 86.

43. Latner, A. L., Molyneux, L., and Rose, J. D.: *J. Lab. & Clin. Med. 43:* 157, 1954.
44. Bower, V. E., Paabo, M., and Bates, R. G.: *Clin. Chem. 7:* 292, 1961.
45. Gambino, S. R.: *Clin. Chem. 7:* 336, 1961.
46. ————: *Clin. Chem. 8:* 199, 1962.
47. O'Mara, T. F., and Faulkner, W. R.: *Am. J. Clin. Path. 33:* 152, 1960.
48. ————, and ————: *Am. J. Clin. Path. 31:* 34, 1959.

3

Collection of Blood and Pipetting

The technic of obtaining blood for ultramicro chemical procedures is a critical step in determinations. It should be the responsibility of the ultramicro technologist or else delegated only to those individuals who have received personal instruction in the technic. Accuracy of the final results is directly dependent on the care with which the samples are obtained from the patients.

Obtaining Capillary Blood

The puncture site should be selected carefully and the technic of collecting the blood sample performed with utmost care since deviation from proper procedures can result in considerable inaccuracy. The site selected is usually the finger tip in an adult and the heel in an infant; either should be cleansed carefully with an alcohol sponge and permitted to dry. The puncture may be made with a sterile Bard-Parker #11 scalpel blade.

The first drop of blood is wiped away gently with sterile gauze. After removing the cap from the collecting tube, a second drop of blood is drawn up into the tube by capillary action. This is accomplished by holding the tube in a nearly horizontal position while touching the drop of blood with the narrow end. Excessive squeezing of the tissues is to be carefully avoided for this will introduce tissue fluids into the sample and may affect accuracy of the results. The blood is allowed to flow down the capillary tube to the larger end without forming bubbles and this end is then capped and the tube returned to the laboratory (*See* Fig. 36).

Collecting Tubes

Samples of blood are obtained in Pyrex capillary tubing with a bore of 1.5-2.7 mm. and an outside diameter up to 4 mm. The tubing is cut into 20 cm. lengths and the central portion is then heated in a gas flame and

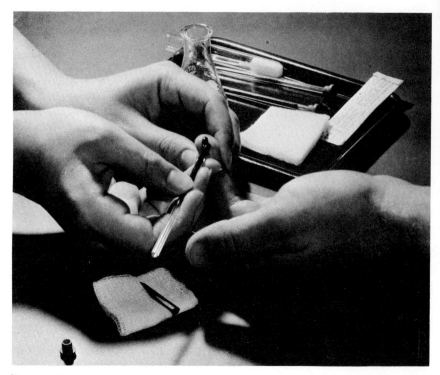

Fig. 36.—Capillary blood is allowed to flow into a nearby horizontal collecting tube. This tube is approximately 9 cm. in length with an outside diameter of 4 mm.

drawn out to a tip suitable for blood sampling. When the tubing is broken in two it provides two sampling tubes. The ends should be fire polished and the tube cleaned carefully and dried before use. Collecting tubes suitable for ultramicro use are also commercially available.*

The wide end of the tube can be sealed off in several ways. Davies[1] suggested the use of a small vaccine vial stopper† and we have found this procedure very satisfactory. Natelson[2] advocates liquid cement; sealing wax or plasticine may also be used. If desired, plastic sealing caps may be purchased.‡

If all determinations are to be performed on serum, no anticoagulant is necessary. If the use of plasma is required, an anticoagulant may be drawn up several times into the capillary tubing and expelled in order to coat the

---

* Micro blood collecting tubes, Scientific Products #51600; blood collecting tubes, Scientific Industries, Inc.

† #68 MS orange V-3 stopper, West Co.

‡ Critocap-K, Scientific Products #51663; disposable clear caps, Scientific Industries, Inc.

walls of the tubing. Directions for the preparation of anticoagulants are included in the chapter on Microhematocrits.

Serum vs. Plasma

Although the use of serum has been most satisfactory for the methods used routinely in our laboratories, it is preferable or even necessary to use plasma in some situations.[3] The use of plasma permits immediate biochemical analysis of the samples after they have reached the laboratory. It minimizes changes in the electrolyte balance of the sample, and rapid testing of plasma samples for glucose also reduces errors resulting from glycolysis.

The use of plasma, on the other hand, is not without its hazards. This is the result of the introduction of foreign substances as anticoagulants. As the anticoagulants are usually available in the form of sodium, potassium, or ammonium salts, the effect of these salts on the accuracy of the determination must always be taken into consideration. The use of plasma containing the sodium salt of heparin for sodium analysis[3] remains open to question. The anticoagulant may also materially affect the analysis of respiratory gases by altering the pH of the sample.[4]

Protection of Sample from Air

Methods have been devised for collecting capillary blood under oil to avoid contact with air for chloride determinations and the analysis of respiratory gases.[5] However, the technical skill required to achieve such sampling is considerable, particularly since this procedure is usually performed on uncooperative infants who take little interest in expediting its accuracy. If the collecting tube is filled with blood and stoppered promptly, there is very little contact with air and there is doubt if the method requiring oil offers a significantly greater degree of accuracy. It may be expedient to substitute the carbon dioxide combining power method drawn in the usual manner.

A very precise method of blood collecting for the analysis of respiratory gases in plasma and whole blood is described by Holaday and Verosky.[6] They use 2 mm. syringes for this purpose. The plunger is coated with light stopcock grease, and the dead space in the syringe is filled with a solution consisting of one part of saturated sodium fluoride solution and 10 parts of heparin solution, 50,000 units per ml. Immediately after obtaining the sample, a droplet of mercury is drawn into the syringe through a fine-bored needle. Subsequent manipulations of the sample are performed anaerobically.

Removal of Serum from Collecting Tubes

To minimize changes in the electrolytes and to prevent hemolysis of the serum sample, the serum should be removed from contact with the cell column as promptly as possible. The capillary tube is filed at the upper end of the serum column and broken off at this point. Sharp separation of serum and clot is achieved by centrifugation. The capillary tube is placed with the stoppered end down in an ordinary table model centrifuge and spun for several minutes. The tube may now be filed and broken at a point just above the junction of serum and clot and the serum tube recapped. Serum may be stored for longer periods of time by the method described by Davies.

The serum (or plasma) is removed by aspiration into an ultramicro pipet, using either the constriction type or one of the overflow varieties.

Alternative Methods of Blood Collection

An alternative method of collecting capillary blood is outlined in the technical bulletin supplied with the Beckman/Spinco ultramicro analytical system.[7] A glass microhematocrit tube is inserted into a plastic micro test tube. The first drop of blood is wiped away; the second drop is allowed to grow large. Holding the micro test tube nearly horizontal, place the mouth of the capillary tube in contact with the drop of blood. Permit the blood to flow in, without air bubbles, until the capillary tube is full. Now turn the micro test tube to a vertical position and allow the blood to run out of the capillary tube into the micro test tube. A flick of the wrist may be necessary to start the blood flowing. After removal of the capillary tube, the blood is ready for centrifugation. If the skin puncture has been of adequate size, the capillary tube can be filled two or three times, giving sufficient serum for multiple determinations. Plastic blood collectors designed by Rasmussen[8] have been used in the laboratory of Hurley Hospital. These blood collectors fit the Misco 1 ml. centrifuge tubes as well as the Spinco and Coleman plastic centrifuge tubes and they should prove useful to those who collect samples directly into these tubes.

Blood collection for pH determinations is so critical to the proper performance of the procedure that its discussion is deferred to the chapter on pH.

REFERENCES

1. DAVIES, J. A. V.: *J. Lab. & Clin. Med. 23:* 1206, 1938.
2. NATELSON, S.: *Am. J. Clin. Path. 21:* 1153, 1951.
3. SAIFER, A., GERSTENFELD, S., AND ZYMARIS, M. C.: *Clin. Chem. 4:* 127, 1958.
4. ROMANSKI, R. N.: Personal communication.
5. DRUCKER, P., AND CULLEN, G. E.: *J. Biol. Chem. 64:* 221, 1925.
6. HOLADAY, D. A., AND VEROSKY, M.: *J. Lab. & Clin. Med. 47:* 634, 1956.
7. BECKMAN/SPINCO TECHNICAL BULLETIN #6070B, 1960.
8. RASMUSSEN, R. F.: Personal communication. *March,* 1962.

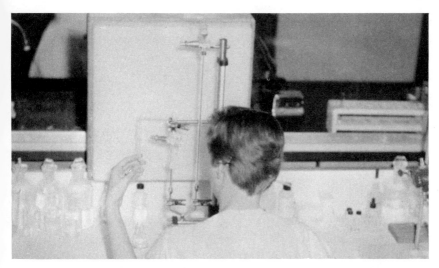

Fig. 37.—Determining carbon dioxide combining power.

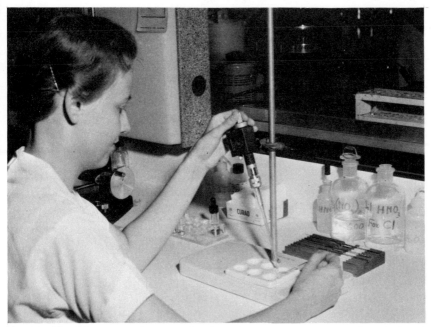

Fig. 38.—The Gilmont pipet-buret may be clamped in position over a spot plate. A digital counter records the amount of reagent expelled, while mixing is performed with a glass stirring rod.

4

Amylase

Principle

Serum alpha-amylase activity is measured by incubating serum with a starch solution buffered at pH 7.5 for 15 minutes. The enzyme activity is stopped with 0.1N hydrochloric acid, and an iodine solution is added to form the blue starch-triiodide ion complex. A control tube is run simultaneously in the same manner as the test sample, except the serum is not incubated with the starch solution. The optical density of both tubes is read in a spectrophotometer at 620 mμ, using a dilute iodine solution as a reagent blank. Amylase activity is determined in Somogyi units (mg. starch degraded/10 ml. serum/30 min.), and the procedure has been adjusted to result in these units. This method follows the technic suggested by Rice[1] in which the starch solution is made stable with sorbic acid and a tris buffer is used.

Apparatus

Pipet, KMP or other ultramicro type, 10 lambdas
Pipet, KMP or other ultramicro type, 50 lambdas
Pipet, KMP or other ultramicro type, 100 lambdas
Pipet, KMP or other ultramicro type, 200 lambdas
Pipet, 0.5 ml. volumetric
Test tubes, 7 x 70 mm.
Volumetric flasks, 2.0 ml. capacity
Water bath, 37 C.

Reagents

1. *Sorbic acid-starch solution:* Prepare a saturated aqueous solution of sorbic acid by adding about 3 Gm. of sorbic acid (obtainable from K & K Laboratories, Long Island City 1, N.Y.) to about 1100 ml. of distilled water and allowing it to stand at room temperature with occasional mixing for

several days before removing the undissolved acid by filtration. Suspend 1.000 Gm. of starch (soluble according to Lintner, Merck, special for diastatic power determination) in approximately 50 ml. of the saturated sorbic acid solution in a liter volumetric flask. Add about 300 ml. of boiling saturated sorbic acid solution three times, mixing well by swirling the flask rapidly after each addition. Cool the solution to room temperature, and dilute to volume with saturated sorbic acid solution. Store the water-clear reagent (pH 3.4) in a polyethylene bottle at room temperature.

2. *Tris buffer, pH 7.5:* Dissolve 19.4 Gm. of tris (hydroxymethyl) aminomethane in about 800 ml. of distilled water. Adjust to pH 7.5 with concentrated hydrochloric acid, and dilute to one liter of water. Tris (hydroxymethyl) aminomethane is available from Distillation Products Industries as 2-amino-2-hydroxymethyl 1,3-propanediol, EK 4833. Tris buffer is recommended instead of a phosphate buffer because it is not subject to mold growth.

3. *Sodium chloride solution, 0.9 per cent:* Dissolve 0.9 Gm. sodium chloride in water and dilute to 100 ml. in a volumetric flask.

4. *Hydrochloric acid solution, 0.5N:* Dilute 42 ml. of concentrated hydrochloric acid to one liter with distilled water.

5. *Stock iodine solution, 0.1N:* Dissolve 30 Gm. potassium iodide in about 250 ml. of distilled water in a liter volumetric flask. Add 13 Gm. of iodine and shake flask until the iodine is completely dissolved. Dilute to volume, and store in a dark bottle in the refrigerator.

6. *Working iodine solution, 0.01N:* Dilute 1 ml. of the stock iodine solution to 10 ml. with distilled water. The solution keeps about one week when stored in a dark bottle in the refrigerator.

Procedure

1. Pipet 200 lambdas 0.9 per cent saline into a 7 × 70 mm. test tube. Add 10 lambdas of serum and mix thoroughly.

2. Into each of two 2 ml. volumetric flasks pipet 100 lambdas of starch solution and 100 lambdas of tris buffer. Label one flask "Test" and the other "Control." Place both flasks in a water bath at 37 C. for 3 to 5 minutes.

3. Add 50 lambdas of diluted serum to "Test" flask, mix well, and incubate in the water bath for *exactly* 15 minutes.

4. At the end of the 15-minute incubation period, stop the reaction by adding 100 lambdas of 0.5N hydrochloric acid solution to both flasks.

5. Add distilled water until both flasks contain about 1.5 ml. of solution.

6. Add 50 lambdas of diluted serum to the "Control" flask.

7. Pipet 50 lambdas of working iodine solution into each flask, and into a third flask labelled "Blank." Dilute to mark with distilled water.

8. Pipet 0.5 ml. of distilled water into each flask, mix thoroughly by inversion, and allow to stand for 5 minutes.

9. Transfer to microcuvets, set the spectrophotometer at 620 mμ wave length, and 100 per cent transmittance with the "Blank" solution. Read the optical density of the solutions in both flasks. The color is stable for several hours.

Calculations

$$\frac{OD \text{ "Control"} - OD \text{ "Test"} \times 800 \times Dilution}{OD \text{ "Control"}} = \text{Units Amylase Activity}$$

$$\text{Dilution Factor for 1:21 dilution} = 1.05$$
$$\text{Dilution Factor for 1:84 dilution} = 4.2$$

If amylase activity of more than 350 Units is found, repeat the test by using a 1:84 dilution (50 lambdas of the 1:21 diluted serum added to 150 lambdas of 0.9 per cent saline).

Normal Values

Adults: 40-160 units
Infants (under 1 year):   5-40 units

Discussion

The determination of serum amylase by use of the blue starch-triiodide ion complex is the most practical ultramicro approach, but it was not previously used because of the difficulty in preparing a stable standard starch solution. The modification proposed by Rice which is used here overcomes this difficulty. Caraway[2] uses benzoic acid as a starch preservative and a phosphate buffer.

Henry and Chiamori[3] report the necessity for an adequate concentration of starch in the substrate. They found that only above a limiting concentration of starch (representing saturation of enzyme with substrate) would a linear reaction rate be observed for a period of time that was directly related to the initial starch concentration. When the enzyme is no longer saturated with starch, deviation from a linear reaction rate occurs, and hydrolysis of lower molecular-weight sugars becomes significant. Rice gives 350 units as the level at which this method must be repeated, using a greater dilution of serum. This should be short of the point at which complete hydrolysis is indicated, i.e., where the "Test" and "Control" solutions give the same reading.

Blood levels of amylase in a normal individual are quite constant and are not affected by diet. The concentration is low during the first two months of life, rising slowly to adult levels by the end of the first year of life.[4] Residual enzyme from the mother's blood causes higher values during the first 3 days after birth.[5]

Acute pancreatitis is rarely seen in childhood, but in adults it is accompanied by a rise in activity of amylase within a few hours with elevated levels persisting 3 to 4 days. Occasional patients with mumps or salivary gland infection have high serum amylase levels.[6] Other causes of elevated amylase activity include perforated peptic ulcer, uremia, methanol poisoning, cholecystitis, and small bowel obstruction. Codeine and morphine can also cause moderate increases.[7] Lower levels can be encountered with necrotizing pancreatitis, hepatitis, severe burns, toxemia of pregnancy and poisoning by barbiturates, arsenic or carbon tetrachloride.

REFERENCES

1. RICE, E. W.: *Clin. Chem. 5:* 592, 1959.
2. CARAWAY, W. T.: *Am. J. Clin. Path. 32:* 97, 1959.
3. HENRY, R. J., AND CHIAMORI, N.: *Clin. Chem. 6:* 434, 1960.
4. EASTHAM, R. D.: Biochemical Values in Clinical Medicine. Bristol, England, John Wright & Sons, Ltd., 1960.
5. SUNDERMAN, F. W., AND BOERNER, F.: Normal Values in Clinical Medicine. Philadelphia, W. B. Sanders, 1950.
6. HOFFMAN, W. S.: The Biochemistry of Clinical Medicine. 2nd Ed. Chicago, Year Book Publishers, 1960.

5

Bilirubin

Principle

The bilirubin in serum is diazotized with Ehrlich's reagent to form azobilirubin. The red-violet color is compared with the color from a standard solution of bilirubin treated in the same manner. The addition of methyl alcohol to the serum permits measurement of the total bilirubin. The use of an aqueous solution measures the "direct" bilirubin, or bilirubin glucuronide. The reagents used here are those suggested by Meites,[7] and result in a higher extinction coefficient and require less time for reaction than the van den Bergh reagents used in the Evelyn and Malloy procedure.[6]

Apparatus

Pipet, KMP or other ultramicro type, 20 lambdas
Pipet, KMP or other ultramicro type, 25 lambdas
Pipet, KMP or other ultramicro type, 100 lambdas
Pipet, KMP or other ultramicro type, 200 lambdas
Pipet, KMP or other ultramicro type, 250 lambdas
Pipet, volumetric, 5 ml.
Pipet, serologic, 0.2 ml.
Test tubes, 7 x 70 mm.

Reagents

1. *Diazo A reagent:* Dissolve 5 Gm. of reagent sulfanilic acid in 60 ml. of concentrated hydrochloric acid, mix, and dilute to one L. with distilled water. Stable indefinitely.

2. *Sodium nitrite, 20 per cent:* Dissolve 20 Gm. of reagent sodium nitrite in distilled water and dilute to 100 ml. Store in a brown glass-stoppered bottle in the refrigerator. Keeps indefinitely, but discard if solution becomes tinged with yellow.

3. *Diazo B reagent:* Dilute the stock 20 per cent sodium nitrite 1:10 (e.g. 0.5 ml. + 4.5 ml. distilled water). Prepare fresh daily.[4]

4. *Diazo blank reagent:* Dilute 60 ml. of concentrated hydrochloric acid to 1 L. with distilled water.

5. *Diazo reagent:* Add 0.15 ml. of (B) to 5 ml. of (A) and mix well. This reagent is stable about 30 minutes.[4]

6. *Stock standard, 20 mg. per cent:* Weigh out exactly 0.200 Gm. bilirubin (see discussion), and transfer to a 100 ml. volumetric flask. Dissolve and dilute to mark with chloroform. Store in a brown bottle in the refrigerator.

7. *Working standard, 2 mg. per cent:* Pipet 10 ml. stock standard into a 100 ml. volumetric flask, dilute to mark with absolute methyl alcohol and mix. Use immediately after preparation.[4]

Procedure

1. **Transfer 25 lambdas of serum into a 7 × 70 mm. test tube. Add 250 lambdas of distilled water and mix thoroughly by gently tapping. This results in a serum dilution of 1:11.**

2. **Pipet 100 lambdas of absolute methanol into a 7 × 70 mm. test tube labelled A (sample) and the same quantity into another tube labelled B (blank).**

3. **Pipet 20 lambdas of *fresh* diazo reagent into tube A and 20 lambdas of diazo blank reagent into tube B.**

4. **Add 100 lambdas of diluted serum to each. Mix by gently tapping and allow to stand at room temperature for 10 minutes.**

5. **Measure transmittancy of the sample and the reagent blank in a Beckman spectrophotometer at 560 mμ. Distilled water is used to set the instrument at 100 per cent transmittance.**

6. **To determine "direct" reacting bilirubin, the same procedure is followed, except that distilled water is substituted for methanol, and the colored solution is read in exactly 5 minutes.**

Calculation

$OD_A - OD_B \times F$ = mg. per 100 ml. bilirubin
    See Calibration for F

Calibration

1. Prepare 5 dilute standards by diluting 1, 2, 3, 5 and 10 ml. of working bilirubin standard to 10 ml. with absolute methanol and mixing thoroughly.

Use within a few minutes after preparation. These standards correspond to bilirubin concentrations of 4.4, 8.8, 13.2, 22.0 and 44.0 mg. per cent, based on the use of 100 lambdas of a 1:11 dilution of the original serum.

2. Pipet 200 lambdas of each diluted standard into five 7 x 70 mm. test tubes. Transfer 200 lambdas methanol to another tube to serve as a reagent blank.

3. Add 20 lambdas of fresh diazo reagent to each and mix by gently tapping. Allow to stand at room temperature for 10 minutes.

4. Measure transmittancy as given under Procedure.

5. Prepare a standard curve by plotting concentration in mg. per 100 ml. against optical density. This will demonstrate conformance to Beer's law over the entire range of values. Calculate the factor (F) for each standard. The average value for all the standards will serve as the factor for the determination of bilirubin in the unknown specimens.

$$F = \frac{\text{Equivalent mg. per 100 ml. bilirubin*}}{\text{OD standard} - \text{OD blank}}$$

Discussion

Blood used for this determination should be free of hemolysis. A decrease of up to 25 per cent in azobilirubin formation has been found to vary directly with the amount of hemolysis.[7] Avoid contaminating the reagent blank with diazo reagent. If the same cuvet is used for both reagent blank and samples, the reagent blank solution should be read first in the spectrophotometer.

Bilirubin determinations should be performed immediately after drawing the specimen since bilirubin is light sensitive. O'Hagan[9] tested the effect of sunlight for one hour (2:45 to 3:45 p.m. on a bright spring day) and found the value dropped from 9.0 mg./100 ml. to 4.8 mg. per 100 ml.

The problem of standards for bilirubin determination has been given much consideration. Discrepancies in standard solutions have long been noted, and these may be caused by either the instability of the standard solutions, or to the bilirubin preparation itself. Carter and McGann[2] tested Fisher, Eastman Kodak and Hoffman-LaRoche products and found all three gave the same spectrophotometric curves over the range 400-700 mμ. They suggested that the cause for discrepancies was failure to consider the instability of the standard solutions. Bilirubin in chloroform-methanol solution is very unstable. Deterioration begins immediately after preparation, and after 30-60 minutes the extinction coefficient at 440 mμ is half its original value. Precipitation of a yellow pigment occurs after several hours, and by 8-12 hours a green tint develops. Deterioration occurs more rapidly in the light than in the dark.

---

* Equivalent based on the 1:11 dilution of serum sample.

Stock chloroform solutions of bilirubin are stable at least 3 months when stored in the dark at 4 C. Dilute sodium nitrite solutions are stable 6 hours, and diazo reagent for about 30 minutes.

The use of sodium carbonate solution as a diluent for bilirubin standards has been suggested.[4, 10] Schellong and Wende[10] dissolve 40 mg. bilirubin in 50 ml. of 0.1 M sodium carbonate, then add 2 ml. of this solution to 13.9 ml. of fresh, normal, fasting serum, followed by 0.1 ml. of 4 N acetic acid. This adds 10 mg. per 100 ml. bilirubin to the bilirubin concentration of the original serum. A second solution is prepared containing 13.9 ml. of the original serum, 2 ml. of 0.1 M sodium carbonate, and 0.1 ml. of 4 N acetic acid. The difference in absorbence obtained from analysis of the two solutions represents that of the added bilirubin.

Henry, Jacobs, and Chiamori recommend a standard of purity for bilirubin preparation.[4] They found only the preparations of Pfanstiehl and Matheson, Coleman and Bell were completely soluble in chloroform; all other commercial products contained some insoluble brown pigment. They suggest checking the *azobilirubin* absorptivity of the commercial product, and if it is not close to that of pure bilirubin (63,500 to 64,600), then either purify the bilirubin, or correct for the absorbency obtained on the standard (A_s).

$$\text{Corrected } A_s = \frac{64,100}{\text{absorptivity obtained}} \times A_s \text{ obtained}$$

The addition of albumin to a pure bilirubin standard does not significantly alter the absorbance of azobilirubin.[7] There is, however, a small but significant decrease in absorbence when albumin is added to serum, but this is important only when the protein concentration exceeds the normal physiologic range. The differences between standardization with serum and chloroform-methanol solutions of bilirubin is probably due to the inhibition of the color reaction by small amounts of chloroform and the 3 per cent decrease in volume occurring when equal volumes of methanol and aqueous solutions are mixed.[4] Since these factors are ordinarily not taken into consideration, Meites reports standardization in methanol gives values 10 per cent higher than the same standards in serum.[8] Results in the test procedure would therefore be lowered by this amount.

Room temperature for this procedure should be in the vicinity of 22-37 degrees.[7] Marked variation in temperature will cause incomplete coupling of the bilirubin.

The procedure described uses the modified van den Bergh reagents proposed by Meites.[7] The absorbence of azobilirubin is increased and the reaction time accelerated to 10 minutes by increasing the concentration of hydrochloric acid, sulfanilic acid, and sodium nitrite.

The total bilirubin is usually of greater pediatric interest than the "direct." The "direct" and "indirect" terminology has been followed for many years following the original hypothesis by van den Bergh. The older rationale for these two reactions has been discussed in many texts, and was always based upon quite questionable evidence. Cole, Lathe and Billing[3] reported in 1955 that the non-polar bile pigment which predominates in the serum of patients with hemolytic jaundice is bilirubin. In 1956 Schmid[11] in the U.S. and Billing and Lathe[1] in England found the water-soluble prompt-reacting fraction of the van den Bergh reaction to be bilirubin glucuronide. Hydrolysis of 1 μM of azo pigment B (direct) with β-glucuronide produced 1 μM of glucuronic acid. Since 1 M of bilirubin produces 2 M of this azo pigment, the direct reacting bilirubin is conjugated with 2 M of glucuronic acid. A small amount may be conjugated as the monoglucuronide, thus satisfying reports of two water soluble fractions. Liver is the site of formation of these conjugates. Excessive destruction of hemoglobin (as in hemolytic anemia) causes an elevation in the indirect fraction. Intrahepatic or extrahepatic obstruction to the passage of bile into the intestine will cause a rise in the direct fraction. The preferred terminology for the van den Bergh reaction would now be *bilirubin* and *bilirubin glucuronide* rather than indirect and direct bilirubin.

Azobilirubin is an acid-base indicator. The differences between various curves reported for the Evelyn and Malloy method may be the result of acidity differences.[2] Stoner and Weisberg[12] made use of a lower pH to determine bilirubin by a diazo blue reaction. Others[5] have demonstrated the absorption maxima depend on the pH. It shifts from 560 in acid solutions to 510-520 in neutral solutions, and back to 570-580 in alkaline solutions.

The normal values usually given for adults do not apply to the newborn, the majority of whom have physiologic hyperbilirubinemia with or without accompanying jaundice. This physiologic elevation is highest between the second and fifth day after birth. The peak in the full-term infant is usually on the second day although it tends to occur later in the premature infants. Hsia et al. in their work on serum bilirubin levels in the newborn infant, point out that a cord bilirubin level over 5 mg. per 100 ml. is strongly suggestive of erythroblastosis.[13, 14] Peak elevation of bilirubin of premature infants not only occurs later than that of full-term infants, but reaches considerably higher levels. Reinhold quotes Lathe in reporting that the serum bile pigment concentration of 8-pound babies is usually less than 3-5 mg. per 100 ml., while that of 4-pound babies is much higher and may rise to 10-15 mg. per ml.[15] Hsia feels that a level of serum bilirubin above 10 mg. per 100 ml. during the first 24 hours of life, or the appearance of visible icterus during this period, must be considered due to erythroblastosis until proved otherwise. Therefore, bilirubin determinations are indispensable in the diagnosis and prognosis of erythroblastosis due either to Rh or ABO incompatibility. The bilirubin should not be allowed to go above 20 mg. per 100 ml. if possible; untreated cases can reach levels of 60-70 mg. per 100 ml.[16]

In the study of hemolytic transfusion reactions, Davidsohn and Stern recommend determination of serum bilirubin and urea nitrogen on pre- and post-transfusion specimens, to be repeated at 24-hour intervals as indicated.[17] Ultramicro studies are particularly valuable in these instances where only limited samples of serum are available.

REFERENCES

1. BILLING, B. H., AND LATHE, G. H.: *Biochem. J. 63:* 6, 1956.
2. CARTER, R. E., AND McGANN, C. J.: *Clin. Chem. 5:* 106, 1959.
3. COLE, P. G., LATHE, G. H., AND BILLING, B. H.: *Biochem. J. 57:* 514, 1955.
4. HENRY, R. J., JACOBS, S. L., AND CHIAMORI, N.: *Clin. Chem. 6:* 529, 1960.
5. JIRSA, M., AND JIRSOVA, V.: *Clin. Chem. 5:* 532, 1959.
6. MALLOY, H. T., AND EVELYN, K. A.: *J. Biol. Chem. 119:* 48, 1937.
7. MEITES, S., AND HOGG, C. K.: *Clin. Chem. 5:* 470, 1959.
8. MEITES, S.: Manual of Clinical Chemistry. The Children's Hospital of Columbus, Ohio, 1960.
9. O'HAGAN, J. E., HAMILTON, T., LE BRETON, E. G., AND SHAW, A. E.: *Clin. Chem. 3:* 609, 1957.
10. SCHELLONG, G., AND WENDE, U.: *Klin. Wchnschr. 38:* 703, 1960.
11. SCHMID, R.: *Science 124:* 76, 1956.
12. STONER, R. E., AND WEISBERG, H. F.: *Clin. Chem. 3:* 22, 1957.
13. HSIA, D. Y. Y., ALLEN, F. H., DIAMOND, L. K., AND GELLIS, S. S.: *J. Pediat. 42:* 277, 1953.
14. HSIA, D. Y. Y., ALLEN, F. H., GELLIS, S. S., AND DIAMOND, L. K.: *New England J. Med. 247:* 668, 1952.
15. REINHOLD, J. G.: *Clin. Chem. 1:* 351, 1955.
16. DIAMOND, L. K., ALLEN, F. H., VANN, D. D., AND POWERS, J. R.: *Pediatrics 10:* 337, 1952.
17. DAVIDSON, I., AND STERN, K.: *Am. J. Clin. Path. 25:* 381, 1955.

6

Calcium

ERIOCHROME BLACK T METHOD

Principle

Calcium in serum is precipitated as the oxalate, dissolved in hydrochloric acid and chelated with an excess of ethylene diamine tetra-acetic acid (EDTA).[1] The excess unchelated EDTA is titrated with a standard magnesium solution in a buffered medium using eriochrome black T as an indicator. Calcium may be calculated by titration of suitable standard calcium solutions.

Apparatus

Pipet, KMP or other ultramicro type, 100 lambdas
Pipet, KMP or other ultramicro type, 200 lambdas
Pipet, volumetric, 1.0 ml.
Test tubes, 10 x 50 mm., 15 x 125 mm.
Ultramicro pipet-buret, Gilmont, 1 ml. capacity
Titration mixing apparatus: Bend a six inch length of glass tubing to a 90° angle and then draw out one end to a fine capillary. Connect to the pipet-buret so that the capillary end extends along the glass tip; the other end is attached to a compressed air supply. A steady stream of air forced into the titration mixture will facilitate determination of the end-point. If no compressed air is available, air blown from the mouth of the operator may be used, but a small flask of glass beads should be used as a baffle to prevent saliva from entering the mixture.

Reagents

1. *Double-distilled water.*
2. *Ammonium oxalate, 3.5 per cent:* Place 3.5 Gm. of reagent quality

ammonium oxalate in a 100 ml. volumetric flask and dissolve with about 50 ml. of double distilled water. Dilute to mark and mix.

3. *Hydrochloric acid, 1N:* Dilute 85 ml. of reagent quality hydrochloric acid to one liter with double-distilled water and mix.

4. *Ethylene diamine tetra-acetic acid, 0.005 M:* Transfer to a 1 liter volumetric flask exactly 1.860 Gm. of reagent quality disodium salt of ethylene diamine tetra-acetic acid. Dissolve and dilute to mark with double-distilled water. (Keeps indefinitely).

5. *Magnesium solution, 0.005 M:* Transfer exactly 1.020 Gm. of reagent quality magnesium chloride ($MgCl_2 \cdot 6H_2O$) to a one-liter volumetric flask. Dissolve and dilute to mark with double distilled water. This is a stock solution; for a working solution dilute 1:1 with double-distilled water.

6. *Buffer solution:* Dilute 70 ml. reagent quality ammonium hydroxide to one liter with double-distilled water. Keep in a well-stoppered bottle.

7. *Indicator solutions:*

Solution A: Dissolve 100 mg. of eriochrome black T and 900 mg. of reagent quality hydroxylamine hydrochloride ($NH_2OH \cdot HCl$) in 20 ml. of reagent quality methanol.

Solution B: Dissolve 50 mg. of methyl red in 100 ml. of 95 per cent ethanol.

Indicator Solution: Mix one part A with two parts B. Prepare this solution only as required, fresh for each day's use.

8. *Calcium Stock Standard Solution (0.4 mg. Ca per ml.):* Dry in a 110-120 C. oven overnight approximately 1.5 Gm. of reagent quality calcium carbonate. Cool in a desiccator and transfer exactly 1.000 Gm. to a one liter volumetric flask. Dissolve in 25 ml. of reagent quality hydrochloric acid. After reaction ceases, dilute to mark with double-distilled water.

Procedure

1. Pipet 200 lambdas of double-distilled water into a 10 × 50 mm. test tube.

2. Add 100 lambdas of serum.

3. Add 200 lambdas of 3.5 per cent ammonium oxalate solution. Mix well by running bottom of tube gently back and forth over a wire test tube rack. Allow to stand at least 5 minutes; the longer the time the more complete the precipitation.

4. Place the 10 × 50 mm. test tube into a 15 × 125 mm. test tube and centrifuge 12-5 minutes in a standard size clinical centrifuge.

5. Discard the supernatant solution by carefully inverting the tube.

6. Add 200 lambdas of 1N HCl and mix well. The precipitate should be completely dissolved.

7.   Add 1.0 ml. of buffer solution, 100 lambdas of EDTA solution, and two drops of indicator solution. Mix.

8.   Titrate with the standard magnesium solution, using an ultramicro pipet-buret and the titration mixing apparatus. The titrate is a greenish-gray color. The end-point is the first appearance of a grayish-pink color.

9.   A reagent blank (*important*) is titrated for each determination. It contains:

> 200 lambdas of 1N HCl
> 100 lambdas of water
> 1.0 ml. of buffer solution
> 100 lambdas of EDTA
> 2 drops of indicator solution

Calculation

The titration reading of the reagent blank minus the sample is used to obtain mg. per 100 ml. calcium directly from the standard curve.

Calibration

1. Prepare five working standards by diluting 1, 2, 3, 4, and 5 ml. of the calcium stock standard solution to 10 ml. These dilutions will be equivalent to 4, 8, 12, 16, and 20 mg. per cent calcium.

2. Using each of the above standards, titrate the following mixture with 0.005M magnesium solution to the grayish-pink color.

> 200 lambdas 1N HCl.
> 100 lambdas diluted Ca standard.
> 1.0 ml. buffer solution.
> 100 lambdas of EDTA solution.
> 2 drops indicator solution.

3. Prepare and titrate a reagent blank as outlined under Procedure.

4. Plot results on plain graph paper. The mg. per 100 ml. calcium will be the abscissa and the corresponding titration value (magnesium solution used for titrating the blank minus amount required for the sample) is the ordinate. The result should be a straight line.

Comment on Method

This rapid method eliminates many of the possible errors of the traditional methods. Uric acid does not interfere and the precipitate need not be washed, since the precipitated calcium is measured indirectly. This ultramicro method will give values agreeing within two per cent of those obtained with the Clark-Collip macro procedure.[2] Extra precautions should be taken in this method to avoid contamination of the glassware. It is best to keep separate test tubes and pipets to be used only for this purpose.

Numerous other modifications of the EDTA chelation have been described. The Spinco system utilizes a calcein indicator with serum samples of 20 lambdas.[3-9] The Coleman ultramicro analysis is a modification of methods of Bachra, Sauer, and Sobel[9] and Meites;[10] it makes use of the Cal-Red indicator.

The presence of large amounts of phosphate (as in urine specimens) will cause the blue color of the end-point to appear before the true equivalence point is reached, due to the precipitation of the calcium as the phosphate at the high pH used for the titration. As precipitated calcium dissociates from the phosphate, the color gradually changes back to the purple pre-equivalence point color. Sodium citrate may be added to complex with the calcium and prevent formation of calcium phosphate; calcium is released as the EDTA is added.

A problem in calcium measurement is the interference by magnesium. Patton and Reeder[11] showed that much of this interference is eliminated by titration at a high pH, where magnesium is quantitatively precipitated as the hydroxide but is not chelated until all free calcium and all calcium bound by the indicator is chelated by the EDTA. Van Schouwenburg has proposed the use of Carbocel to eliminate the interference of magnesium in EDTA titrimetric procedures, with murexide as the indicator.[12]

CORINTH CALCIUM METHOD*

Principle

This method, described by Yangisawa,[13] utilizes a purple dye (disodium 1-hydroxy 4-chloro 2, 2-diazobenzene 1, 8-dihydroxynaphthalene-3, 6-disulfonic acid) which becomes red in the presence of calcium.

Magnesium does not interfere if the reaction is carried out in a strongly alkaline solution.[14]

Apparatus

Pipet, KMP or other ultramicro type, 20 lambdas

---

* As modified by James S. Brush, Ph.D., formerly of the Department of Pathology, Hurley Hospital, Flint, Mich.

Pipet, KMP or other ultramicro type, 250 lambdas

Flasks, volumetric, 25 ml.

Pipet, 2ml., graduated 0.1 mil. 1 Test tubes, 1 ml. "Misco"

Reagents

1. *Stock dye 0.035 M:*   Weigh 46.0 mg. of Corinth calcium (disodium 1-hydroxy-4-chloro 2, 2-diazobenzene-1, 8-dihydroxynaphthalene-3, 6-disulfonic acid) into a 25 ml. volumetric flask. Add 0.25 ml. of 0.03N HCl, dilute to volume with distilled water. Keep this reagent in refrigerator. (Corinth calcium can be purchased from Clinton Laboratories, 6010 Wilshire Boulevard, Los Angeles 36, Calif.)

2. *0.03N HCl:*   Dilute 2.5 ml. of concentrated HCl (sp. gr. 1.18) to one liter with water.

3. *Alkaline dye solution:*   Add 1.0 ml. of stock dye solution to a 25 ml. volumetric flask and dilute to volume with 10N NaOH. Prepare fresh before use.

4. *1.0N NaOH:*   Since sodium hydroxide is not very pure, containing much carbonate, it is advisable to buy commercially made 10N NaOH solution and dilute it to the desired normality.

Take 10 ml. of 10N NaOH solution and dilute it to 100 ml. with water.

5. *Stock standard calcium:*   Dry 2 Gm. of reagent grade calcium carbonate overnight at 110-120 C. Cool in dessicator and weigh 1.2511 Gm. of it into a glass stoppered Erlenmeyer flask. Add 2.5 ml. concentrated reagent grade HCl slowly to flask, being careful to avoid spattering of contents out of flask. Transfer contents quantitatively to a one liter volumetric flask and dilute to volume. (1 ml. = 0.025 mEq. calcium.)

Procedure

Using a 250 lambda KMP pipet twice, transfer 0.5 ml. aliquots of alkaline dye solution into well-washed 1 ml. Misco tubes. Add 20 lambdas of serum, standard and distilled water to these tubes, rinsing the pipet with the alkaline dye solution. Mix the solution well before reading. Transfer solutions into clean Beckman micro cells. Set wave length at 635 mμ. Read the optical density of each solution, setting the instrument to 10 per cent transmission with the alkaline dye solution.

Standardization

Prepare three 25 ml. volumetric flasks as follows: Make about 100 ml. of one molar calcium chloride solution. Fill the 25 ml. volumetric flasks to the top with the calcium chloride solution. Allow to stand for several hours, discard solution and rinse flasks four to five times with distilled water. Then add 7 ml. of stock standard calcium solution to the 25 ml. volumetric flasks, rinsing the pipets used twice in stock standard before using. (These procedures are necessary to insure that no calcium is lost to glass surfaces, thereby lowering the amount of calcium measured.) These dilutions contain 7 mEq./L. of calcium.

Run 20 lambdas of this standard along with the serum to determine the standard curve.

Calculation

$$\text{Ca content in unknown (mEq./L.)} = \frac{(\text{O.D. blank} - \text{O.D. unknown}) \times 7}{\text{O.D. blank} - \text{O.D. standard}}$$

$$\text{O.D. blank} = 1.000$$

Notes

Capillary and venous blood obtained at the same time were analyzed for Ca. There was no difference in the Ca values.

One sample of serum was taken and analyzed 15 times for Ca. Difference between the highest value (5.55 mEq./L. Ca) the average value (5.40 mEq./L. Ca) and the lowest value (5.26 mEq./L. Ca) found was ± 2.7 per cent.

Pooled serum was analyzed for Ca. Known amounts of Ca were added. 93.9, 100.0 and 103.0 per cent of added Ca was recovered.

COLEMAN FLAME PHOTOMETER

Principle

See Chapter 22.

Apparatus

Pipet, KMP or other ultramicro type, 200 lambdas
Pipet, KMP or other ultramicro type, 100 lambdas
Volumetric flask, 5 ml.
Micro sample container, Coleman 21-310

Reagents

1. *Sterox solution, 1 per cent:* Weigh 5.0 Gm. (± 0.1 Gm.) of Sterox SE in a tared 250 ml. beaker. Add about 200 ml. of distilled water and mix.

Transfer quantitatively into a 500 ml. volumetric flask. (When diluting or using Sterox solutions, run the solution down the side of the flask to prevent excessive foaming.) Dilute with distilled water to the mark and mix. Store in a polyethylene bottle.

2. *Sodium, 6.0 mEq./L., and Sterox 0.02 per cent:* Pipet 12.0 ml. of standard reagent A (See Chapter 22, p. 183) into a 500 ml. volumetric flask. Add 10.0 ml. of reagent 1 and dilute to mark with distilled water. Mix well. Store in a polyethylene bottle.

3. *Sterox, 0.02 per cent:* Pipet 10 ml. of reagent 1 into a 500 ml. volumetric flask. Dilute to mark with distilled water and mix. Store in a polyethylene bottle.

4. *Lab-Trol or Versatol.*

Procedure

1.   Place 1-2 ml. of distilled water in a 5 ml. volumetric flask. Set up one extra flask for the Lab-Trol standard.

2.   Add 100 lambdas of reagent 1 to each flask.

3.   Pipet 200 lambas of serum of Lab-Trol into each flask. If possible, perform all analyses in duplicate.

4.   Dilute to 5 ml. mark with distilled water. This is a 1:25 dilution of the serum.

5.   Pour into micro sample containers.

6.   Place Ca filter in slot and push down firmly. Set steadiness control at 10 and Galv. Coarse control at about 1.

7.   Place a beaker containing reagent 2 in the sample carrier of the flame photometer, close the door and atomize sample. Set galvanometer at zero with BLK control on flame photometer.

8.   Replace this beaker with a beaker containing diluted Lab-Trol standard. Adjust scale reading to calcium value of Lab-Trol, using GALV knobs on the galvanometer.

Note: Scale reads in mEq./L. of calcium. mEq./L. × 2 = mg. per cent Ca. Therefore a Lab-Trol Ca of 10 mg. per cent is 5 mEq./L., and the 5 should be set on the scale panel. In reading unknowns, multiply scale values by 2 to convert to mg. per cent.

9.   Flush with reagent 3 each time after aspirating a sample containing serum or Lab-Trol.

10.   Repeat steps 7 and 8 until constant readings are obtained.

11.   Aspirate and read values of unknowns.

12.   The Coleman autoflow system may also be used with this procedure.

Note: Lab-Trol or Versatol are recommended as standards because, in the authors' experience, pooled frozen serum specimens give erratic calcium values. Aqueous standards are not recommended and will not give reliable results.

Many flame photometers may be adapted for use in calcium determinations. The very high flame temperatures and high photodetector sensitivity required for calcium increase the amount of background and radiation interference, however. The serum phosphate particularly is a source of radiation interference.[16, 20, 24] Interfering substances of high concentration may be added to both unknowns and standards[15] to improve the accuracy by providing a more constant background. Internal standards[17] may be used to compensate for varying fuel pressure, fluid flow and instrument sensitivity, but they will not correct for the relatively high physiologic concentration of sodium and phosphate.

CAL-RED METHOD

Calcium in serum is determined by titration against a standard solution of EDTA (ethylenediamine tetra acetic acid) in an alkaline solution. When all the calcium has been chelated by the EDTA, the Cal-Red indicator changes from wine-red to blue. The color of the end-point of each titration is compared to the previously titrated specimen.

Apparatus

Micrometric syringe microburet or Gilmont pipet-buret, capacity 1 ml.
Lab-jack, Cenco-Lerner (if syringe microburet is used)
Pipet, KMP or other ultramicro type, 50 lambdas
Pipet, KMP or other ultramicro type, 100 lambdas
Pipet, 0.5 volumetric
Spot plate

Reagents

1. *Potassium hydroxide, 1.25 N:* Dissolve 70 Gm. 85 per cent KOH in water and dilute to one liter. Standardize this solution by titration against a standard acid. Store in a polyethylene bottle.

2. *EDTA solution, 0.93 Gm./L.:* Weigh exactly 0.93 Gm. disodium ethylenediamine tetra acetic acid, transfer to a one liter volumetric flask, and dilute to mark with distilled water. Store in a pyrex or polyethylene bottle.

3. *Cal-Red solution:* Weigh 100 mg. Cal-Red [2-hydroxy-1-(2-hydroxy-4-sulfo-1-naphthylazo)-3-naphthoic acid] (obtainable from Scientific Service Laboratories Inc.) and dilute to 100 ml. with distilled water. This solution will keep 3 weeks in the refrigerator.

4. *Caprylic alcohol.*

5. *Sodium cyanide solution, 1 per cent:* Dissolve 1.0 Gm. sodium cyanide in 100 ml. distilled water.

6. *Lab-Trol or Versatol.*

Procedure

1. Transfer a 100 lambda sample of Lab-Trol in duplicate to a spot plate depression. Add 1 drop of caprylic alcohol.

2. Add 0.5 ml. of KOH solution to each, and also to each of two adjacent depressions to serve as a blank.

3. Add 50 lambdas of Cal-Red solution to the blank solutions and immediately titrate with EDTA. *Note:* Do not add indicator solution to more than two samples at one time because the color fades rapidly.

4. Add 50 lambdas Cal-Red solution to the standard samples and titrate to the same color as the blank samples.

5. The unknown samples are titrated in the same manner as the standards, adding indicator only before immediate use, and using the prior titration as a reference in each case. The color change is from wine-red to blue. It may help to look for the absence of the purple color. The end-point will be green in the case of hemolyzed serum.

6. In solutions containing iron or copper, a drop of cyanide solution is added prior to the titration.

Calculation

$$\frac{\text{Volume of EDTA titrated for sample}}{\text{Volume of EDTA titrated for standard}} \times \frac{\text{Ca concentration}}{\text{in standard}} = \frac{\text{mg. per 100 ml.}}{\text{Ca in sample}}$$

Note: The color of the end-point observed in titrating a standard containing protein is more directly comparable to that observed with the unknown serum. Therefore Lab-Trol or Versatol are recommended rather than aqueous standards. In the authors' experience, pooled frozen serum specimens are not reliable as calcium standards.

Comment on Method

This procedure is highly reproducible except in hemolyzed or icteric serum, when the end-point is somewhat obscured.

Normal Values (Serum Calcium)

Newborn: 7.5-13.5 mg. per 100 ml.
Infants: 10.5-12 mg. per 100 ml.
Children: 10-11.5 mg. per 100 ml.
Adults: 9-11 mg. per 100 ml.
        4.5-5.7 mEq./L.

Discussion

Serum protein levels influence the calcium level since approximately one-half of the calcium is present in a non-diffusible form bound to serum proteins. If the total protein concentration is known, the level of free calcium ions may be calculated by use of the McLean-Hastings nomogram.[30] From a pediatric standpoint, measurement of calcium ions in children with hypoproteinemia or hyperproteinemia shows the true state of calcium distribution in the serum. Altered levels of protein may mask an altered level of calcium.

In general there is a reciprocal relation between calcium and phosphorus levels. However, the older Ca × P product is no longer considered entirely valid for diagnostic purposes.

Calcium levels are lowered in uremia, severe nephritis, hypoparathyroidism, tetany, renal rickets, pregnancy, acute pancreatic necrosis, nephrosis, pneumonia, osteomalacia and sprue. Calcium is elevated in hyperparathyroidism, in carcinoma metastatic to bone, in multiple myeloma, and after fractures.

REFERENCES

1. REHELL, R.: Scandinav. J. Clin. & Lab. Invest. 6: 335, 1954.
2. CLARK, E. P., AND COLLIP, J. B.: J. Biol. Chem. 63: 461, 1925.
3. DIEHL, H., AND ELLINGBOE, J. L.: Anal. Chem. 28: 882, 1956.
4. BIEDERMANN, W., AND SCHWARZENBACH, G.: Chimia 2: 56, 1948.
5. SCHWARZENBACH, G., AND ACKERMANN, H.: Helvet, Chim. Acta 30: 1798, 1947.
6. _____, ANDREGG, G., FLASCHKA, H., AND SALLIMAN, R.: Helvet. Chim. Acta 37: 113, 1954.
7. _____, BIEDERMANN, W., AND BANGERTER, F.: Helvet. Chim. Acta 29: 811, 1946.
8. _____, AND GYSLING, H.: Helvet. Chim. Acta 32: 1314, 1949.
9. BACHRA, B. N., SAUER, A., AND SOBEL, A.: Clin. Chem. 4: 107, 1958.
10. MEITES, S.: Manual of Clinical Chemistry. Columbus, Ohio, The Children's Hospital of Columbus, 1959.
11. PATTON, J., AND REEDER, W.: Anal. Chem. 28: 1026, 1956.
12. VAN SCHOUWENBURG, J. CH.: Anal. Chem. 32: 709, 1960.
13. YANAGISAWA, F.: J. Biochem. 42: 3, 1955.
14. KINGSLEY, G. R., AND ROBNNET, O.: Am. J. Clin. Path. 27: 223, 1957.
15. AHRENS, L. H.: Spectrochemical Analysis. Cambridge, Mass., Addison-Wesley Press, 1950.

16. BAKER, G. L., AND JOHNSON, L. H.: *Anal. Chem. 26:* 465, 1954.
17. BERRY, J. W., CHAPPELL, D. G., AND BARNES, R. C.: *Ind. Eng. Chem., Anal. Ed. 18:* 19, 1946.
18. BRABSON, J. A., AND WILHIDE, W. D.: *Anal. Chem. 26:* 1060, 1954.
19. CARAWAY, W. T., AND FANGER, H.: *Am. J. Clin. Path. 25:* 317, 1955.
20. CHEN, P. S., JR., AND TORIBARA, T. Y.: *Anal. Chem. 25:* 1642, 1953.
21. DENSON, J. R.: *J. Biol. Chem. 209:* 233, 1954.
22. KAPUSCINSKI, V., MOSS, N., ZAK, B., AND BOYLE, A. J.: *Am. J. Clin. Path. 22:* 687, 1952.
23. KINGSLEY, G. R., AND SCHAFFERT, R. R.: *Anal. Chem. 25:* 1738, 1952.
24. MOSHER, R. E., ITANO, M., BOYLE, A. J., MYERS, G. B., AND ISERI, L. T.: *Am. J. Clin. Path. 21:* 75, 1951.
25. POWELL, F. J. N.: *J. Clin. Path. 6:* 286, 1953.
26. ROTHE, C. F., AND SAPIRSTEIN, L. A.: *Am. J. Clin. Path. 25:* 1076, 1955.
27. SEVERINGHAUS, J. W., AND FERREBEE, J. W.: *J. Biol. Chem. 187:* 621, 1950.
28. VON SCHULTZ, G. L.: *Schweiz. med. Wchnschr. 83:* 333, 1953.
29. WINER, A. D., AND KUHNS, D. M.: *Am. J. Clin. Path. 23:* 1259, 1953.
30. MCLEAN, F. C., AND HASTINGS, A. B.: *J. M. Sc. 189:* 601, 1935.
31. BRUSH, J. H.: *Anal. Chem. 33:* 798, 1961.

7

Carbon Dioxide Combining Power

Principle

Carbon dioxide is usually measured by acidification of the sample and manometric or volumetric determination of the liberated gas. It may also be measured titrimetrically. Acid may be added to liberate the carbon dioxide present and the excess acid titrated, or barium carbonate may be precipitated, washed, and titrated.[1]

The instrument most widely used at the present time for ultramicro carbon dioxide determinations is the Natelson manometric Van Slyke apparatus.[2, 3] Natelson, using at first a volumetric type of Van Slyke instrument, found the volume of the liberated bubble of gas constantly decreases with time; this is the result of redissolving of the carbon dioxide brought to atmospheric pressure after liberation under a vacuum. Thus, unless readings are taken quickly, results are erroneous.

The Natelson microgasometer, requiring only 0.03 ml. of serum, measures the CO_2 gas manometrically under constant volume. As originally described by Natelson, only the gas soluble in alkali (3 N sodium hydroxide) was measured. This method is theoretically the most accurate and certainly would be required if the blood contained nitrous oxide, ether, or other gases used in general anesthesia. Descriptions are available in Natelson's book on microtechnics[1] or in Caraway's *Microchemical Methods for Blood Analysis.*[4]

A shorter method, however, has been found more satisfactory for routine use, particularly as the alkali is very difficult to clean from the machine. This method utilizes the relative constancy of the serum gases other than carbon dioxide, and, by omitting the alkali absorption step, eliminates the difficulties with the sodium hydroxide. A calibration curve is constructed to determine the factor necessary to compensate for omitting the alkali absorption step.

PROCEDURE 1

Apparatus

> Microgasometer, Natelson, Model 600 (shaker attachment and illuminated background optional) (See Fig. 37, p. 55)
> Pipet, KMP or other ultramicro type, 50 lambdas
> Centrifuge tube, 1 ml.
> Reagent bottles, screw-cap, supplied with apparatus
> "Equilibrating bottle"

Note: A small bottle of 50-100 ml. capacity is filled with glass beads and stoppered with a 2-hole rubber stopper. Two pieces of glass tubing are bent to right angles and inserted into these holes. One tube (air inlet) extends to the bottom of the bottle and the other (air outlet) just above the surface of the glass beads. Rubber tubing is attached to each piece of glass tubing and capillary tube is placed at the end of the outlet tubing. The glass beads should be cleaned and dried monthly.

Reagents

Lactic acid, 1 N: Dilute 9 ml. of reagent quality 85 per cent lactic acid to 100 ml. with distilled water and mix.

Carbon dioxide standard solution (25 mEq./L.): This solution may be used for practicing technic and for checking the method. Dry about 3 Gm. reagent quality anhydrous sodium carbonate overnight in a 100-120 C. oven. Cool in a desiccator and weigh out exactly 2.650 Gm. Transfer to a one-liter volumetric flask, dissolve and dilute to mark with distilled water. Store in a glass-stoppered pyrex bottle and place a thin layer of mineral oil over the solution to prevent air absorption.

Reagent vials: The following reagents should be layered in reagent vials:

Vial #1	Mercury		Vial #2	Mercury
	Lactic acid			Distilled water
	Caprylic alcohol			

Procedure

1. Transfer 50 lambdas or more, but not more than 100 lambdas, serum to a 1 ml. centrifuge tube and equilibrate with alveolar air using the equilibrating bottle. Direct the stream of air at the top of the serum with constant mixing. Spread serum over the wall of the tube during equilibration. Repeat at least twice and analyze without delay. Keep the centrifuge tube stoppered with a fingertip between equilibrations.

2. Advance mercury in the gasometer until a small drop is held on the tip of the pipet.

3. Draw 0.03 ml. of equilibrated serum into the microgasometer. Wipe pipet tip with clean tissue or gauze.

4. From vial #1 introduce in the following order:

      0.01 ml. mercury

      0.03 ml. lactic acid

      0.01 ml. mercury

      0.01 caprylic alcohol

      0.01 ml. mercury

These reagents are layered in the vial so that the mercury is at the bottom, lactic acid in the middle and caprylic alcohol at the top. Wipe pipet tip with clean gauze or tissue. Keep the tip of the pipet in the center of the vial when introducing reagents. It is convenient to rest the left elbow on the bench top and to hold one finger against the pipet to steady the vial.

5. Introduce from vial #2, 0.10 ml. of distilled water, then mercury to the 0.12 mark on the reaction chamber. Wipe off the pipet tip.

6. Close the reaction chamber stopcock and retreat the piston until the mercury is at the 3.0 ml. mark. Raise the mercury level until there is a small bead of mercury in the reaction chamber. If mercury remains in the section of the reaction chamber below the stopcock, briskly turn the stopcock a little to one side, then to the other. *Caution!* Do not open stopcock.

7. Loosen the shaker screw knob on the base of apparatus and shake for one minute by grasping hand wheel firmly and swinging apparatus back and forth in short arcs.

8. Bring aqueous meniscus to 0.12 mark and record pressure reading (P_1) and temperature.

9. Advance piston until mercury is at the top of the manometer, open reaction chamber stopcock and advance mercury until all aqueous matter is out of the instrument. (*Caution:* Place the waste bottle under the pipet tip.)

10. Rinse twice with distilled water drawing the water into the reservoir under the reaction chamber. (*Caution:* Do not introduce any air when rinsing the instruments.) Expel all aqueous matter.

11. Introduce from vial #2

      0.03 ml. water and

      0.01 ml. mercury

12. Introduce from vial #1 in the following order:

      0.03 ml. lactic acid

0.01 ml. mercury

0.01 ml. caprylic alcohol

0.01 ml. mercury

13. Introduce from vial #2, 0.10 ml. distilled water, then mercury to the 0.12 mark on the reaction chamber.

14. Close the reaction chamber stopcock and retreat the piston until the mercury is at the 3.0 ml. mark.

15. Proceed as in steps 6 and 7 and record the pressure reading (P_2).

Calculation

$$(P_1 - P_2) \times F = \text{mEq./L. } CO_2 \text{ Combining Power}$$

F (temperature factor) is supplied with apparatus and calculated by means of basic gas laws and certain corrections for incomplete extraction and re-absorption of CO_2.

Note: It is possible to further simplify this procedure by omitting steps 10-15. In this modification, after completing step 9, close manometer stopcock, retreat mercury meniscus to 0.12 mark and use this manometer reading as the P_2. If this procedure is followed, carry out the following calibration procedure.

Calibration

To calculate new factors for CO_2 estimation for the modified method, the Van Slyke and Neill equation[4] and Van Slyke and Sendroy data[5] can be used. It is simpler, and for clinical purposes accurate enough, to cross-calibrate the microgasometer with a conventional Van Slyke manometric apparatus.

Collect several specimens of serum or plasma with high, normal, and low CO_2 combining powers. Samples on either extreme may be prepared by adding 20 lambdas (microliters) 2N sodium carbonate or 2 N hydrochloric acid to 3 ml. of normal serum. Equilibrate these samples with alveolar air, transfer under oil to a small test tube and analyze CO_2 combining power on the conventional Van Slyke manometric apparatus. Immediately analyze the same sample with the microgasometer using the shortened procedure. Calculate the F (factor) for the new procedure as follows:

$$\frac{CO_2 \text{ content in standard sample}}{P_1 - P_2} = F$$

These factors usually fall very close to the factors given with the Natelson microgasometer on a given temperature.

If the CO_2 estimation factors supplied with the instrument are used with the shorter method, the following correction should be made:

$$(P_1 - P_2 - C) \times F = CO_2 \text{ content in unknown, where}$$

$P_1 = P_{CO_2} + P_{O_2} + P_{N_2} + P_{H_2O} + P$ misc. gases which are released from serum and reagents

$P_2 = P_{O_2} + P_{N_2} + P_{H_2O} + P$ misc. gases which are released from distilled H_2O used as serum blank to replace the volume and reagents

C represents the difference between the pressure of gases liberated from distilled water and from serum, expressed in terms of the reading on the micro-gasometer. This constant value may then be used for all subsequent determinations. For routine clinical use this correction is negligible and may be ignored.

PROCEDURE 2

In this alternate procedure,[9] two non-ionic polyols replace the caprylic alcohol used in procedure 1. There is less contamination of the glassware, and the instrument requires less frequent cleaning.

Reagents

1. *Lactic acid, 1 N:* Same as procedure 1.

2. *Carbon dioxide standard solution, 25 mEq./L.:* Same as procedure 1.

3. *Low foam detergent, 0.5 per cent:* Dilute 10 ml. of reagent No. 810 (Scientific Industries) to 100 ml. with distilled water.

4. *Anti-foam, 10 per cent:* Use the 10 per cent solution as purchased (Reagent No. 820, Scientific Industries). Shake well.

5. *Reagent Vials:* Prepare the following reagent vials:

        Vial #1 Lactic acid, 1 N.
                  mercury
        Vial #2 Anti-foam reagent
                  mercury
                  (Shake the vial before each use)
        Vial #3 Low-foam detergent
                  mercury

Procedure

1. Same as procedure 1.

2. Advance the mercury in the gasometer until a small drop is held on the tip of the pipet.

3. Draw 0.03 ml. of equilibrated serum into the microgasometer. Wipe pipet tip with clean tissue or gauze.

4. From vial #1 introduce in the following order:

        0.01 ml. mercury

        0.03 ml. lactic acid

        0.01 ml. mercury

Wipe pipet tip with clean gauze or tissue. Keep the tip of the pipet in the center of the vial when introducing reagents. It is convenient to rest the left elbow on the bench top and to hold one finger against the pipet to steady the vial.

5. Introduce from vial #2:

        0.01 ml. Anti-foam reagent

        0.01 ml. mercury

Wipe pipet tip as before.

6. Introduce from vial #3:

        Low-foam detergent to the 0.1 ml. mark

        Mercury to the 0.12 ml. mark on the reaction chamber

        Wipe off pipet tip.

7. Continue, beginning with step 6 in Procedure 1.

Normal Values

Adults: 25-32 mEq/L.

        55-70 vols. per 100 ml.

Children: 18-25 mEq./L.

        40-55 vols. per 100 ml.

Discussion

This ultramicro method will show good agreement with the classic Van Slyke technic when calibrated as described. The accuracy of this simplified procedure is well within the error usually allowed for clinical procedures. Reproducibility is very good. Any slight deviations are usually due to the equilibrating technic rather than the method of analysis.

The carbon dioxide content of serum as measured manometrically includes dissolved carbon dioxide gas, carbonic acid, and bicarbonate ion. If the pH is normal, the major part of the total carbon dioxide is bicarbonate; thus total carbon dioxide provides a practical estimate of the bicarbonate present. The capillary tube method of blood collecting permits very little exposure of the collected serum to air, and if the carbon dioxide content is measured promptly there appears to be relatively little advantage in collecting the specimen under oil. Also, chance introduction of oil into the system is a disadvantage of the latter method. The spun cells and serum should be separated promptly. For situations where maximum accuracy is required, methods for collecting small blood samples under oil are described in the literature.[1, 6, 7]

Carbon dioxide combining power determinations are satisfactory for most of the types of cases where ultramicro methods are required, as it is much more common in infants to be dealing with situations involving metabolic alkalosis. Of course the re-equilibration may introduce errors if the partial pressure of the alveolar carbon dioxide differs in patient and technologist.

Another type of microgasometric apparatus has been developed by Lazarow.[8] This instrument is equipped with a magnetic stirring device and a dial indicator gauge.

Neither the Beckman/Spinco nor the Coleman ultramicro packages provide reliable methods for measuring carbon dioxide combining power or content, a rather serious deficiency when one considers that one of the major indications for ultramicro procedures is the measurement of electrolyte values in children and in burn cases. The titrimetric method proposed by Beckman/Spinco has not been found reliable.[10]

REFERENCES

1. NATELSON, S.: Microtechniques of Clinical Chemistry for the Routine Laboratory. Springfield, Ill., Charles C Thomas, 1957, pp. 147-152.
2. NATELSON, S.: *Am. J. Clin. Path. 21:* 1153, 1951.
3. CARAWAY, W. T., AND FANGER, H.: *Am. J. Clin. Path 25:* 317, 1955.
4. CARAWAY, W. T.: Microchemical Methods for Blood Analysis. Springfield, Ill., Charles C Thomas, 1960, p. 65.
5. VAN SLYKE, D. D., AND SENDROY, J., JR.: *J. Biol. Chem. 73:* 127, 1927.
6. MACDONALD, R. P.: *J. Michigan M. Soc. 55:* 538, 1956.
7. KAPLAN, S. A., AND DEL CARMEN, F. T.: *Pediatrics 17:* 857, 1956.
8. LAZAROW, A.: *Lab. Invest. 2:* 22, 1953.
9. Instruction Suppl. #1, Natelson Microgasometer, Scientific Industries, Inc., Springfield, Mass.
10. O'BRIEN, D., IBBOTT, F., AND PINFIELD, A.: *Clin. Chem. 7:* 521, 1961.

8

Cephalin Flocculation Test

Principle

This is an ultramicro modification of the Hanger cephalin flocculation test.[1] The flocculation is believed to be caused by serum gamma globulin and in normal serum this flocculation is inhibited by substances in the albumin fraction.[2] Normally a balance exists, but pathologically there may be an increase in the gamma globulin fraction or a decrease in the albumin fraction so that there is insufficient albumin component to inhibit the flocculation reaction. No difference has been found between albumin from serum which gives a positive reaction and albumin from serum which does not.[3]

Apparatus

Pipet, KMP or other ultramicro type, 10 lambdas
Pipet, KMP or other ultramicro type, 50 lambdas
Pipet, KMP or other ultramicro type, 200 lambdas
Test tubes, 6 × 50 mm.

Reagents

1. *Sodium chloride, 0.9 per cent:* Transfer 0.9 Gm. sodium chloride to a 100 ml. volumetric flask, dissolve in distilled water and dilute to mark.

2. *Cephalin-cholesterol antigen:*

(a) Cephalin-cholesterol mixture: This consists of 100 mg. of partially oxidized cephalin and 300 mg. of cholesterol. The cephalin may be prepared by dehydrating and extracting sheep brain but it is much simpler and more satisfactory to purchase it. One commercial antigen (Wilson & Co., Inc.) has been shown to give fewer positive results for both normal people and patients with non-liver disorders while retaining sensitivity for detecting patients with liver damage.[4]

(b) Stock solution: Dissolve the dry cephalin-cholesterol mixture in 8 ml. of ether (U.S.P., anesthesia). This stock solution is stable if kept tightly stoppered in the refrigerator.

(c) Working antigen solution: Warm 18 ml. of freshly distilled water to 65-70 C. and add to this 0.5 ml. of stock ether solution. Heat to boiling and continue boiling gently until final volume is 15 ml. Cool to room temperature in the dark. This emulsion must be prepared fresh each day.

Procedure

1. Pipet 10 lambdas of serum into a 6 × 50 mm. test tube. Label another 6 × 50 mm. test tube *Blank*.

2. Add 200 lambdas of 0.9 per cent NaCl and 50 lambdas of working antigen solution to each tube. Mix contents of both tubes thoroughly.

3. Stopper with cotton and allow to stand undisturbed at room temperature *in the dark*.

4. Read after 24 hours in the following manner:[5]

Neg. = Milky solution with no visible flocculation

1+ = Evenly dispersed and faint precipitate seen clearly only when tube is held to the light.

2+ = Heavier precipitate than 1+ but completely dispersed.

3+ = Heavy precipitate partially settled to bottom of tube with supernatant still cloudy.

4+ = Complete flocculation, leaving supernatant clear.

Normal Values

24 hours = Negative

48 hours = Negative to 2+

Discussion

Clean glassware must be used to avoid contamination from acids, heavy metals or bacteria. If the serum is refrigerated one day or more, false positive reactions will result. Neither the serum nor the test solution should be exposed to light from any source. It is also important to prepare fresh working antigen every day.

The conventional method for reading cephalin flocculation tests is used here. Quantitative methods have been developed using either the degree of clearing[6] or the amount of cholesterol in the precipitate.[7] The cephalin flocculation test is positive in active parenchymal liver disease. In acute viral hepatitis the test will be positive soon after the onset of the disease, even before an elevation of serum bilirubin. Negative results do not preclude viral hepatitis however.[8] Positive tests may or may not continue during the recovery period.

The test in this book is also positive in cirrhosis, pneumonia, malaria and infectious mononucleosis, and is useful in prognosis of hepatitis patients. Negative reactions before a reduction of the icterus gives a favorable indication. Prolonged positive results with dropping or unchanged icterus indicate progressive liver degeneration.

REFERENCES

1. HANGER, F. M.: *J. Clin. Invest. 18:* 261, 1939.
2. MOORE, D. B., PIERSON, D. S., HANGER, F. M., AND MOORE, D. H.: *J. Clin. Invest. 24:* 292, 1945.
3. CHARLWOOD, P. A.: *Biochem. J. 56:* 480, 1954.
4. KATZ, E. J., HASTERLIK, R. J., AND SNAPP, F. E.: *J. Lab. & Clin. Med. 44:* 353, 1954.
5. HEPLER, O. E.: Manual of Clinical Laboratory Methods, 4th Ed. Springfield, Ill., C. C Thomas, 1952.
6. KILBRICK, A. C., RODGERS, H. E., AND SKUPP, S. J.: *Am. J. Clin. Path. 22:* 698, 1952.
7. JENNINGS, E. R., CHERNEY, P., AND ZAK, B.: *Am. J. Clin. Path. 23:* 1173, 1953.
8. NEFFE, J. R., GAMBESCIA, J. L., GARDNER, H. L., AND KNOWLTON, M.: *Am. J. Med. 5:* 600, 1952.

9

Chlorides: Serum and Spinal Fluid

MERCURIC NITRATE TITRATION

Principle

Serum is titrated directly with a standard mercuric nitrate solution using diphenylcarbazone as an indicator. The mercuric and chloride ions combine without forming a precipitate. Mercuric chloride is undissociated; an excess of mercuric ions at the end point of the titration forms a violet-blue complex salt with diphenlycarbazone. The amount of mercuric nitrate required is a direct measure of the chloride present.

Apparatus

Pipet, KMP or other ultramicro type, 20 lambdas
White porcelain spot plate
Ultramicro pipet-buret, Gilmont, capacity 1 ml.
(*See* Fig. 38, p. 55.)

Reagents

1. *Nitric acid, 0.03 N:* Dilute 2 ml. concentrated reagent quality nitric acid to 1,000 ml. with distilled water and transfer part to a dropping bottle.

2. *Indicator solution:* Dissolve 50 mg. of s-diphenyl carbazone (Eastman) in 50 ml. of 95 per cent ethanol. Store solution in a brown dropping bottle in the refrigerator. The solution should be reddish-orange in color; exposed to light it turns pale yellow and should be discarded. Prepare fresh each month since solutions older than one month fail to give a sharp end point.

3. *Mercuric nitrate solution, 0.01 N:* Transfer 0.81 Gm. reagent quality mercuric nitrate, $Hg(NO_3)_2$, to a 500 ml. volumetric flask. Add 100 ml. of distilled water containing 2 ml. of concentrated nitric acid and mix to dissolve. Dilute to 500 ml. with distilled water, mix again and adjust to 0.01 N against the NaCl standard. The mercuric nitrate solution may be left in the pipet-buret

since the fluid does not come in contact with metal. The pipet-buret is filled in the following manner: The plunger is extended into the glass reservoir and the pipet tip is placed below the surface of the solution to be used. Solution is brought up into the reservoir by retracting the plunger. Entrapped air is removed by inverting the apparatus and allowing the liquid to fall toward the plunger. The plunger is then screwed back into the reservoir until all air has been removed. The entire procedure is repeated until the solution fills the apparatus and no entrapped air remains in the solution. (Further directions for the use of the Gilmont micropipet-buret will be found accompanying the apparatus.)

4. *Sodium chloride standard, 100 mEq./L.:* Dry at least 1 Gm. of reagent quality NaCl overnight in a 110-120 C. oven and cool in a desiccator. Weigh out exactly 0.5845 Gm. of this salt, transfer to a 100 ml. volumetric flask and dilute to mark with distilled water. This keeps indefinitely.

Procedure

1.   Transfer 20 lambdas of serum to a depression on a white porcelain spot plate. If possible, the pipet should be rinsed once with serum to avoid contamination from chlorides in the water. Place 20 lambdas of Lab-Trol in an adjacent depression on the same plate. (See Discussion.)

2.   Add 4 drops of 0.03 N nitric acid to each.

3.   Add 3 drops indicator solution to each.

4.   Titrate with mercuric nitrate standard solution using a Gilmont ultramicro pipet-buret (Fig. 40). Stir with a small glass stirring rod while titrating. The tip of the pipet-buret should be placed at the side of the depression so that it just touches the surface of the liquid at the beginning of the titration. Avoid touching the spot plate, as a fingerprint will greatly elevate the chloride value.

5.   A reagent blank is titrated in the same manner, except that the addition of serum is omitted.

6.   The end-point is the first appearance of a faint blue-violet color.

Calculation

$$\frac{\text{Sample} - \text{blank}}{\text{Standard} - \text{blank}} \times F = \text{mEq./L. serum chloride}$$

$$F = \frac{\text{Titration of Serum Std.}}{\text{mEq./L. chloride in Serum Std.}}$$

mEq./L. chloride $\times$ 5.85 = mg. per 100 ml. serum chloride

Normal Values

Serum	*Sweat*
98 − 106 mEq./L. serum chloride	10 − 60 mEq./L.
570 − 620 mg. per 100 ml.	

Discussion

Values obtained from this ultramicro modification of the Schales and Schales[1] method for the serum chloride agree within 1 per cent of those from the macro technic. Ten replicate analyses on the same serum specimen averaged 98.8 ± 1.2 mEq./L. The macro procedure gave a result of 98.5 mEq./L. Samples obtained simultaneously from a venipuncture and capillary blood showed no significant difference in serum chloride content. Anrode reported that chloride in capillary serum is approximately 1 mEq./L. higher than venous serum.[17] The same procedure is utilized by both the Spinco and Coleman ultramicro systems with very reproducible results.

If necessary, the procedure may be carried out on smaller quantities of serum. Ten lambdas of serum, four drops of 0.03 N nitric acid, and three drops of indicator solution may be used and compared with 10 lambdas of standard serum.

The use of an aqueous standard solution of sodium chloride will tend to produce higher serum values.[18] This is believed to be due to the binding of mercuric ions by the serum proteins. Inclusion of proteins in the standard as recommended here will eliminate these differences between the standard and sample titrations. Any serum may be used as a standard provided the chloride has been determined by other than a direct mercurimetric titration. Icteric serum may still cause difficulty in visualizing the end-point. In this case, the technic of Rice may be used, in which a small amount of ethyl ether is added to the mixture before titration.[19]

Chloride should be determined within 30 minutes after the blood is drawn to prevent the chloride shift from the cells into the plasma. Bromide will titrate against mercuric nitrate in the same manner as chloride so that the titration of serum from patients with bromide poisoning will represent the sum of the chloride plus bromide present.

Gyllensward and Josephson report chloride levels at birth are higher than those in adults, rise for 3 months, and decrease slowly until age 3 years (see Table 3).[20] They believe the high standard deviations they found were due to different stages of development of the infant. Spivek found an arithmetic mean chloride level of 106 mEq./L. in 31 determinations performed on 5-day old normal infants.[2]

Table 3.—Serum Chloride Levels at Different Ages[20]

Age	New-born	3 mo.	6 mo.	(In mEq./L.) 9 mo.	12 mo.	18 mo.	3 yr.	6 yr.	Adult
Mean	107.7	113.6	108.8	108.6	107.8	103.5	101.1	103.4	103
S. D.	8.14	15.2	14.2	13.0	13.5	16.5	9.3	9.7	2.5

Alterations occur through loss of chloride in stomach contents, retention or loss of carbon dioxide, ketosis, kidney disorders, or potassium deficiency alkalosis. Alterations in the concentration of either chloride or bicarbonate is associated with a reciprocal change in the other factor. When chloride is lost in gastric contents there is a compensatory increase in bicarbonate. Primary carbon dioxide retention decreases chloride levels while a carbon dioxide deficit (as in hyperventilation) increases the chlorides. Conditions which raise the level of other serum acids, such as ketosis or renal insufficiency (phosphate retention) may decrease serum chloride as well as bicarbonate. Chloride is increased in nephritis or nephrosis with ammonium chloride therapy.

Increased attention to the diagnosis of cystic fibrosis of the pancreas has made it imperative for many laboratories to develop methods for quantitative analysis of chloride in sweat; ultramicro methods are particularly useful in this respect. The screening tests for electrolytes are most meaningful as negative tests;[3, 4] however, positive screening tests always carry the need for verification by quantitative methods.[5] Values for sodium in sweat above 80 mEq./L. have been found definitive in about 98 per cent of cases,[6] chloride above 60 mEq./L. has been considered diagnostic also when accompanied by relevant clinical data.[7, 8]

Many other approaches to chloride measurement are described in the literature. Cotlove, Trantham and Bowman recommended an electrometric titration with silver ion.[9] For this they use a specially designed instrument providing a constant direct current passing between a pair of silver generator electrodes in the generator (coulometric) circuit. Silver ions are released into the titration solution at a constant rate, and the end-point is indicated after all chloride has been precipitated by the increasing concentration of free silver which causes a rising current to flow through a pair of silver indicator electrodes and a meter-relay in the indicator (amperometric) circuit. At a pre-set level of current an activated relay stops a timer; the amount of chloride precipitated is proportional to the elapsed time. This method is said to be capable of accurately measuring as little as 0.25 mEq. of chloride.

Sanz[10] has combined the bimetallic electrode system of Cunningham, Kirk, and Brooks[11] with the electrode system of Clark.[12] He uses a silver electrode, and, as a reference electrode, the system $Hg/Hg_2SO_4/K_2SO_4$ saturated. This produces a relatively high potential difference which can be measured on a normal valve potentiometer with a sensitivity of 1-2 millivolts.

Spivek's method is the addition to serum of an acid protein precipitate plus a small amount of silver iodate, with formation of relatively insoluble silver chloride.[2] After spinning in a centrifuge, an aliquot of the supernatant is added to a solution of potassium iodide. The iodate which has been displaced by the chloride releases iodine from the potassium iodide, and the resulting color is measured in a photoelectric colorimeter and compared to that produced by a standard chloride solution.

Gibson and Cooke, after using pilocarpine by iontophoresis to produce localized sweating, measure the chloride by polarographic means by a modification of the method of Zimmerman and Layton.[13, 14] Baginski et al. describe three indirect procedures for the quantitative determination of chloride in micro and ultramicro samples. These include polarography by an internal standard method and two absorptiometric procedures exchanging chloride for anions of silver dithizonate or mercuric chloranilate with liberation of dithizone of chloranilic acid.[21]

Another rapid, sensitive chloride procedure is the precision null-point potentiometric method of Malmstadt and Winefordner.[15] Measurements of chloride in samples containing only 0.02 ml. of serum can be carried out in less than 1 minute with an error said to be less than 0.5 per cent. Potentiometric titration methods are also described in detail by Willard, Merritt and Dean,[16] and by Kirman, Morgenstern and Feldman.[22]

Titrations with potentiometric endpoint detection undoubtedly are very useful under certain circumstances, but the mercuric nitrate titration is both rapid and accurate and has proven very satisfactory as a routine ultramicro procedure. Apparently this is also the experience of van Haga and de Wael, who state that the Schales and Schales method can be done with nearly the same accuracy, reproducibility, standard deviation, and speed as the potentiometric titrations.[23]

Whatever method is chosen, it must be kept in mind that changes in the carbon dioxide concentration of the serum lead to a shift of chloride from plasma to erythrocytes or in the opposite direction. Thus, prolonged standing will cause an increased serum chloride content if significant amounts of carbon dioxide have escaped. For this reason serum should be separated rapidly from the cells to avoid a shift from serum to erythrocytes incident to the formation of acid which occurs in the blood upon standing.

SPINAL FLUID CHLORIDE

Chloride in cerebrospinal fluid may be determined as outlined under the method of serum chloride. However, it is best to use the aqueous sodium chloride standard for comparison, due to the relatively small amounts of protein in spinal fluid. Normal values will be 25 per cent higher than for serum chloride, ranging from 720 to 750 mg. chloride per 100 ml. cerebrospinal fluid.

REFERENCES

1. SCHALES, O., AND SCHALES, S. S.: *J. Biol. Chem. 140:* 879, 1941.
2. SPIVEK, M. L.: *J. Pediat. 48:* 581, 1956.
3. SHWACHMAN, H., AND GAHM, N.: *New England J. Med. 255:* 999, 1956.
4. KNIGHTS, E. M., JR., BRUSH, J. S., AND SCHROEDER, J.: *J. A. M. A. 169:* 1279, 1959.
5. DI SANT'AGNESE, P. A., AND ANDERSEN, D. H.: *Ann. Int. Med. 50:* 1321, 1959.
6. BARBERO, G. J.: *Pediatrics 24:* 658, 1959.
7. FINCH, E.: *J. Clin. Path. 10:* 270, 1957.
8. PETERSEN, E. M.: *J. A. M. A. 171:* 87, 1959.
9. COTLOVE, E., TRANTHAM, H. V., AND BOWMAN, R. L.: *J. Lab. & Clin. Med. 51:* 461, 1958.
10. SANZ, M. C., AND BRECHBUHLER, T.: *Rec. trav. chim. Pays-Bas 74:* 531, 1955.
11. CUNNINGHAM, B., KIRK, P. L., AND BROOKS, S. C.: *J. Biol. Chem. 139:* 11, 1941.
12. CLARK, W.: *J. Chem. Soc.* 749, 1926.
13. GIBSON, L. E., AND COOKE, R. E.: *Pediatrics 23:* 545, 1959.
14. ZIMMERMAN, W. J., AND LAYTON, W. M., JR.: *J. Biol. Chem. 181:* 141, 1949.
15. MALMSTADT, H. V., AND WINEFORDNER, J. D.: *Clin. Chem. 5:* 284, 1959.
16. WILLARD, H. H., MERRITT, L. L., JR., AND DEAN, J. A.: Instrumental Methods of Analysis. New York, D. Van Nostrand Co., 1960.
17. ANRODE, H. G, AND MCCRORY, W. W.: *Clin. Chem. 2:* 278, 1956.
18. ANNINO, J. S.: *J. Lab. & Clin. Med. 38:* 161, 1951.
19. RICE, E. E.: *Am. J. Clin. Path. 28:* 694, 1957.
20. GYLLENSWÄRD, C., AND JOSEPHSON, B.: *Scandinav. J. Clin. & Lab. Invest. 9:* 21, 1957.
21. BAGINSKI, E. S., WILLIAMS, L. A., JARKOWSKI, T. L., AND ZAK, B.: *Am. J. Clin. Path. 30:* 559, 1958.
22. KIRMAN, D., MORGENSTERN, S. W., AND FELDMAN, D.: *Am. J. Clin. Path. 30:* 564, 1958.
23. VAN HAGA, P. R., AND DE WAEL, J.: Advances in Clinical Chemistry, Vol. 4. New York, Academic Press, 1961.

10

Total Cholesterol

LIEBERMANN-BURCHARD REACTION

Principle

Total cholesterol is determined by the Liebermann-Burchard reaction. Cholesterol is separated by glacial acetic acid from the globulins to which it is bound and measured by the color developed after addition of acetic anhydride and sulfuric acid.

Apparatus

Pipet, KMP or other ultramicro type, 10 lambdas
Pipet, KMP or other ultramicro type, 20 lambdas
Pipet, KMP or other ultramicro type, 50 lambdas
Pipet, KMP or other ultramicro type, 200 lambdas
Pipet, KMP or other ultramicro type, 500 lambdas
Micro centrifuge tube, 1 ml.
Test tubes, 7 x 70 mm.

Reagents

1. *Acetic acid, glacial, reagent quality.*
2. *Acetic anhydride, reagent quality.*
3. *Sulfuric acid, concentrated, reagent quality.*
4. *Stock cholesterol standard, 200 mg./100 ml.:* Weigh 0.2000 Gm. reagent quality dry cholesterol and transfer to a dry 100 ml. volumetric flask. Dissolve by gently warming in glacial acetic acid and dilute to mark. This standard may be obtained prepared (Hartman-Leddon Co.).
5. *Lloyd reagent, powdered:* (Hartman-Leddon Co.)

Procedure

1. Pipet 20 lambdas of serum into a 1 ml. centrifuge tube.
2. Add 50 lambdas of glacial acetic acid. Mix by gentle tapping and allow to stand at room temperature for about 5 minutes.
3. Add 500 lambdas of acetic anhydride. Mix well and centrifuge for 10 minutes.
4. Place 10 lambdas of concentrated sulfuric acid into a 7 × 70 mm. test tube.
5. Add 200 lambdas of the clear supernatant (3) and mix *immediately*.
6. Allow to stand at room temperature for 15 minutes.
7. Read the optical density *without delay* in a Beckman Spectrophotometer at 680 mμ. Use distilled water to set the instrument at 100 per cent transmittance.
8. A reagent blank may be substituted for distilled water but the difference is usually negligible.

Calculation

OD sample $\times$ F = mg. per 100 ml. total serum cholesterol
   See Calibration for F.

Calibration

1. Pipet 0.4 ml. distilled water into each of seven 50 ml. Erlenmeyer flasks.
2. Add 1.0, 0.9, 0.8, 0.6, 0.4, 0.2, and 0.0 ml. of glacial acetic acid to each.
3 Add stock cholesterol standard solution to each to make a total volume of 1.0 ml., or 0.0, 0.1, 0.2, 0.4, 0.6, 0.8, and 1.0 ml.
4. Add 10 ml. acetic anhydride to each flask and mix. These dilute standards correspond to serum cholesterol concentrations of 0, 50, 100, 200, 300, 400 and 500 mg. per 100 ml.
5. Pipet 10 lambdas of concentrated sulfuric acid into each of the seven 7 x 70 mm. test tubes.
6. Add 200 lambdas of the dilute standard (4) to each and mix.
7. Allow to stand at room temperature and continue with Step 7 under Procedure.

Procedure

$$\text{Factor (F)} = \frac{\text{Equivalent mg. per 100 ml. cholesterol}}{\text{OD Standard}}$$

A calibration curve should be plotted to determine the extent of its linearity. The mean of the F values may be used for calculating daily determinations.

Normal Values

Adults: 140-250 mg./100 ml. cholesterol in serum
Cord Blood:[1] Mean—79.4 mg./100 ml. cholesterol in serum; standard deviation—15.2 mg./100 ml.

Discussion

This method will give values which agree with the Bloor method up to 400 mg./100 ml.[2]

For higher values it is best to dilute serum 1:1 by using 10 lambdas of serum plus 10 lambdas of distilled water.

The patient need not be fasting nor in a basal state when the blood is drawn.[3] Bilirubin will interfere however, and if the specimen appears icteric Lloyd reagent should be added after the acetic anhydride. It should be mixed thoroughly with a small glass stirring rod.

FERRIC CHLORIDE METHOD

Principle

Cholesterol reacts with ferric chloride in the presence of sulfuric acid to produce a purple color.[4-6]

Apparatus

Pipet, KMP or other ultramicro type, 10 lambdas
Pipet, KMP or other ultramicro type, 100 lambdas
Pipet, KMP or other ultramicro type, 150 lambdas
Ultramicro centrifuge tubes, 1 ml.
Flasks, 100 ml. volumetric (2)

Reagents

1. *Cholesterol stock standard, 200 mg./100 ml.:* Dissolve 200 mg. of pure dry cholesterol in glacial acetic acid in a 100 ml. volumetric flask, diluting to mark with glacial acetic acid. This is stable at room temperature.

2. *Ferric chloride stock reagent:* Dissolve 840 mg. ferric chloride ($FeCl_3 \cdot 6H_2O$) in glacial acetic acid in a 100 ml. volumetric flask. Dilute to volume with glacial acetic acid and store in a refrigerator.

3. *Ferric chloride precipitating reagent:* Dilute 2.5 ml. of the stock ferric chloride solution to 25 ml. with glacial acetic acid. Store in a glass-stoppered bottle in the refrigerator.

4. *Ferric chloride diluting reagent and blank:* Dilute 8.5 ml. ferric chloride stock reagent to 100 ml. with glacial acetic acid. Refrigerate.

5. *Concentrated sulfuric acid.*

6. *Glacial acetic acid.*

Procedure

1. Three ultramicro centrifuge tubes are marked *unknown, blank,* and *standard.*

2. Pipet 10 lambdas of serum into the *unknown tube,* 10 lambdas of cholesterol standard into the *standard* tube, and 10 lambdas of distilled water into the *blank* tube.

3. Add 300 lambdas ferric chloride precipitating solution to the *unknown.* Mix well and centrifuge.

4. Add 300 lambdas ferric chloride diluting solution to the *blank* and *standard* tubes. Mix well and let stand 3 minutes.

5. Three more centrifuge tubes are now labeled *unknown, blank,* and *standard* and 150 lambdas supernatant are now transferred from the respective tubes into the clean centrifuge tubes.

6. Carefully layer 100 lambdas concentrated sulfuric acid in each tube. Mix well by tapping tube and let tubes cool to room temperature.

7. Read the optical density of the unknown, standard and blank against distilled water in Beckman DU at 560 mμ.

Calculation

$$\frac{(\text{O.D. unknown}-\text{O.D. blank})}{(\text{O.D. standard}-\text{O.D. blank})} \times 200 = \text{mg./100 ml. cholesterol}$$

Discussion

The method of analysis supplied with the Spinco analytical system is similar to the Caraway-Fanger procedure.[2] Coleman's total cholesterol determination is a modification of Zak's method, in which precipitation of the total proteins is followed by the development of color with ferric chloride in an acid solution.[4-6] Bromide interference may be counteracted by the addition of a small amount of silver iodate,[7] or by using an ion-exchange resin.[14]

Cholesterol levels in plasma are regulated by the liver, which acts as the site of origin and later removes and converts it to cholate (bile acid). Changes in the absorption or excretion of cholesterol have only a moderate effect on the plasma level. Therefore, alterations which occur are due to changes in the rate of synthesis or destruction. Ninety per cent or more of plasma cholesterol is bound to lipoproteins.

Serum cholesterol remains at a fairly constant level for a given individual even though there is a wide range of normal values. A deviation from this constant level in a given person may be pathologically significant even though the cholesterol continues to fall within the normal range of values. Cholesterol levels rise from birth to middle age and then decline slightly. The rise in later middle age however does not always occur. Sex has no effect other than the higher cholesterol level in pregnancy.

Dietary cholesterol as such does not effect serum cholesterol even in large amounts, but the total fat content of the diet does have a marked effect.[8] This effect of diet appears more in middle age. Increased fat content in the diet will cause a rise in serum cholesterol within a few weeks, but it will increase only slowly thereafter.

Severe liver disease causes marked hypocholesteremia, mostly in the esterified fraction. If the liver is only slightly damaged, hypercholesteremia may occur, especially if there is biliary obstruction.

Cholesterol levels are elevated in hypothydroidism but not necessarily lowered in hyperthyroidism.[9] Serum cholesterol is occasionally reduced in anemia, chronic malnutrition, idiopathic steatorrhea and severe infectious diseases.[10] It is elevated in biliary obstruction whether it is caused by calculus, tumor or inflammatory stricture. In intrahepatic biliary obstruction, cholesterol rises if there is no severe necrosis or damage to the liver. Cholesterol is seldom elevated in portal cirrhosis but may be primary biliary cirrhosis. Levels of serum cholesterol rise in severe diabetes with acidosis due to the utilization of lipids from body stores. They are elevated in renal disease if albuminuria, hypoproteinemia or edema are present.

Other cholesterol methods requiring only ultramicro quantities of blood are described in the literature. Galloway et al.[11] have adapted the method of Sperry and Webb to a modification using 40 lambdas of serum to determine both free and total cholesterol. Carpenter, Gotsis and Hegsted[12] report a method involving the measurement of the fluorescence developed after the addition of sulfuric acid to a solution of cholesterol in a mixture of 1,1,2-trichloroethane and acetic anhydride. This is based on the analytical procedure for tissue described by Albers and Lowry[13] and requires 20 lambdas of serum. The variability in results among the various cholesterol methods is considerable, and if the laboratory is to retain a "macro" technic it will be necessary to adopt a matching ultramicro method to avoid confusion.

REFERENCES

1. SOHAR, E., BOSSAK, E. T., WANG, C. I., AND ADLERBERG, D.: *Science 123:* 461, 1956.
2. CARAWAY, W. T., AND FANGER, H.: *Am. J. Clin. Path. 25:* 317, 1955.
3. KEYS, A., ANDERSON, J. T., AND MICKELSON, O.: *Science 123:* 29, 1956.
4. ZLATKIS, A., ZAK, B., AND BOYLE, A. J.: *J. Lab. & Clin. Med. 41:* 486, 1953.
5. ZAK, B., DICKENMAN, R. C., WHITE, E. G., BURNETT, H., AND CHERNEY, P. J.: *Am. J. Clin. Path. 24:* 1307, 1954.
6. ————: *Am. J. Clin. Path. 27:* 583, 1957.
7. RICE, E. W., AND LUKASIEWICZ, D. B.: *Clin. Chem. 3:* 160, 1957.
8. KEYS, A., ANDERSON, J. T., FIDANZA, F., KEYS, M. H., AND SWAHN, B.: *Clin. Chem. 1:* 34, 1955.
9. PETERS, J. P., AND MAN, B.: *J. Clin. Invest. 29:* 1, 1950.
10. BYERS, S. O., FRIEDMAN, M., AND ROSENMAN, R. H.: *Metabolism 1:* 479, 1952.
11. GALLOWAY, L. S., NIELSON, P. W., WILCOX, E. B., AND LANTZ, E. M.: *Clin. Chem. 3:* 226, 1957.
12. CARPENTER, K. J., GOTSIS, A., AND HEGSTED, D. M.: *Clin. Chem. 3:* 233, 1957.
13. ALBERS, R. W., AND LOWRY, O. H.: *Anal. Chem. 27:* 1829, 1955.
14. CHIAMORI, N., AND HENRY, R. J.: *Am. J. Clin. Path. 31:* 305, 1959.

11
Glucose

NELSON-SOMOGYI METHOD

Principle

Zinc sulfate and barium hydroxide are used to prepare a protein-free filtrate of serum which contains only small amounts of reducing substances other than glucose. The glucose in this filtrate is measured by the color formed from the reduction of the cupric ion in an alkaline copper reagent treated with an arseno-molybdate reagent. The color produced is compared with that obtained from a standard solution containing a known amount of glucose. The addition of sodium sulfate to the alkaline copper reagent inhibits reoxidation of cuprous oxide and permits use of plain test tubes.

Apparatus

Pipet, KMP or other ultramicro type, 25 lambdas
Pipet, KMP or other ultramicro type, 50 lambdas
Pipet, KMP or other ultramicro type, 100 lambdas
Pipet, KMP or other ultramicro type, 250 lambdas
Centrifuge tubes, micro, 1 ml.
Test tubes, 7 x 70 mm.

Reagents

1. *Copper reagent, solution A:* Transfer 25 Gm. of anhydrous sodium carbonate (Na_2CO_3), 25 Gm. of Rochelle salt ($NaKC_4H_4O_6 \cdot 4\ H_2O$), 20 Gm. of sodium bicarbonate ($NaHCO_3$) and 200 Gm. of anhydrous sodium sulfate (Na_2SO_4) to a one-liter volumetric flask. Add about 800 ml. of distilled water and mix to dissolve. Dilute to mark, mix, and filter if necessary. Store in a polyethylene bottle in an area where the temperature will not fall below 20 C.

A sediment may form on standing which may be removed by filtration without harm to the reagent.

2. *Copper reagent, solution B:* Transfer 75 Gm. of copper sulfate ($CuSO_4 \cdot 5 H_2O$) to a 500 ml. volumetric flask. Dissolve in distilled water and dilute to mark. Add 0.25 ml. of concentrated sulfuric acid.

3. *Alkaline copper reagent:* Pipet 0.4 ml. of solution *B* into a 10 ml. mixing cylinder and dilute to volume with solution *A*. Mix well. *Prepare fresh daily.*

4. *Arsenomolybdate reagent:* Transfer 50 Gm. of ammonium molybdate, $(NH_4)_6Mo_7O_{24} \cdot 4 H_2O$, to a two-liter Ehrlenmeyer flask, add about 900 ml. distilled water and mix to dissolve. Add 42 ml. of concentrated sulfuric acid (Caution!) and mix. Then add 6 Gm. of disodium orthoarsenate, $Na_2HAsO_4 \cdot 7 H_2O$, dissolved in 50 ml. of water. Mix and incubate for 24-48 hours at 37 C. Formation of a bright yellow precipitate indicates decomposition of the reagent. Store in a brown glass-stoppered bottle.

5. *Zinc sulfate, 5 per cent:* Dissolve 50 Gm. of zinc sulfate, $ZnSO_4 \cdot 7 H_2O$ in distilled water and dilute to one liter in a volumetric flask.

6. *Barium hydroxide, 0.3 N:* Dissolve 45 Gm. of barium hydroxide, $Ba(OH)_2 \cdot 8 H_2O$ in water and dilute to one liter in a volumetric flask. Filter if cloudy. Store in a tightly stoppered polyethylene bottle filled to capacity.

Solutions 5 and 6 should be adjusted so that they neutralize each other. Pipet 10 ml. of $ZnSO_4$ solution into a 250 ml. Ehrlenmeyer flask, add approximately 50 ml. of distilled water and 4 drops of phenolphthalein indicator solution. Titrate slowly with Ba $(OH)_2$ solution with constant mixing. The appearance of a faint pink color indicates the end-point. A false end-point will result if the titration is carried out too rapidly. The 10 ml. aliquot of the $ZnSO_4$ requires 10 ml. ± 0.05 ml. of $Ba(OH)_2$ for neutralization. Adjust the stronger of the two solutions and repeat the titration. The $Ba(OH)_2$ must be stored in an aspirator bottle containing a soda-lime tube in the stopper. Draw this solution from the bottle only as immediately required. Discard the reagent if appreciable amounts of carbonate are formed in the solution.

7. *Benzoic acid, 0.2 per cent:* Transfer 1 Gm. benzoic acid, C_6H_5COOH, to a 500 ml. volumetric flask, dissolve in distilled water and dilute to mark.

8. *Stock standard glucose solution:* Transfer 0.500 Gm. dry glucose to a 500 ml. volumetric flask and dilute to mark with 0.2 per cent benzoic acid. This solution keeps indefinitely.

9. *Working standard glucose solution (25 mg. per cent):* Pipet 25 ml. of stock standard glucose solution into a 100 ml. volumetric flask and dilute to mark with 0.2 per cent benzoic acid.

Procedure

Preparation of the Protein-Free Filtrate:

1. Place 200 lambdas of distilled water in a 1 ml. centrifuge tube.
2. Pipet 20 lambdas serum into the water. Rinse by drawing up solution and expelling it once or twice if a "to contain" pipet is being used.
3. Add 100 lambdas 0.3 N Ba(OH)$_2$ solution and mix by gently tapping.
4. Add 100 lambdas 5 per cent ZnSO$_4$ solution and mix thoroughly by running base of tube gently back and forth over a wire test tube rack, or by use of a mixer.
5. Allow to stand for 3-5 minutes and centrifuge for 3 minutes in a micro centrifuge.

Analysis for Glucose:

6. Transfer 50 lambdas of clear filtrate to a 7 × 70 mm. test tube. Into another tube labelled *blank*, place 50 lambdas of distilled water.
7. Add 100 lambdas of alkaline copper reagent, mix well and stopper loosely. Heat in a boiling water bath for exactly 20 minutes. (*Note:* Water *must* be vigorously boiling!) Transfer to a cold water bath and cool 1-2 minutes.
8. Add 100 lambdas of arsenomolybdate reagent to each tube. Mix thoroughly by running base of tube gently back and forth over a wire test tube rack or by use of a mixer. *When effervescence stops, add 250 lambdas of distilled water and mix by inversion.*
9. Read the optical density on a Beckman DU spectrophotometer at 540 mμ wavelength, using distilled water to set the instrument at 100 per cent transmittance. (*Note:* Check carefully for air bubbles in the cuvet.)

Calculation

OD sample—OD blank × F = mg. per 100 ml. glucose
See calibration procedure for F.

Calibration

1. Prepare 6 glucose standard solutions by diluting 1.0, 2.0, 3.0, 4.0, 5.0 and 10.0 ml. working standard glucose solution to 10 ml. with 0.2 per cent benzoic acid and mixing well. These standards correspond to serum glucose

concentrations of 52.5, 105, 157.5, 210, 262.5 and 525 milligrams per cent based on a 1:21 dilution of the original serum.

2. Transfer 50 lambdas of each dilute standard to a 7 x 70 mm. test tube, and place 50 lambdas of distilled water into another tube labeled blank.

3. Add 100 lambdas alkaline copper reagent to each.

4. Continue as under *Procedure*.

5. Calculate the factor (F) for each dilution by using the following formula:

$$F = \frac{\text{Equivalent mg. per 100 ml. glucose}}{\text{OD standard—OD blank}}$$

The average value is used as the factor for daily determinations. Plot a graph of optical density against equivalent serum glucose concentrations to determine adherence to Beer's law.

Normal Values

Adults: 80-120 mg. per 100 ml. glucose in serum.

Children: 70-120 mg. per 100 ml. glucose in serum.

Note: These values are given for serum. Whole blood values will be between 65 and 110 mg. per 100 ml. In the fasting state the glucose concentrations in capillary and venous serum will be about the same; after ingestion of glucose or food, capillary serum will show higher glucose levels than venous serum.[1]

Discussion

This is an ultramicro modification of the Nelson-Somogyi method[30, 31] which measures "true" glucose rather than total reducing substances. The difference in the levels found in whole blood and serum is due to the smaller amount of intercellular glucose compared to that found in plasma.

The use of sodium sulfate in the alkaline copper reagent inhibits reoxidation of the cuprous oxide permitting use of plain test tubes rather than the constricted tubes required in other methods. The use of the 7 x 70 mm. tube is recommended, however, since they result in a minimum surface area of liquid exposed to air compared to the total volume of the mixture. The final color is stable and will remain unchanged for at least 24 hours. The determination should be performed immediately after blood is drawn to prevent glycolysis.

MODIFIED FOLIN-WU METHOD

Principle

Glucose in a Folin-Wu tungstic acid filtrate is measured by the blue color formed from the reduction of the cupric ion in Somogyi's alkaline copper reagent treated with phosphomolybdic acid. The Somogyi alkaline copper solution is required because of the oxidation which may result from the relatively large surface area in the ultramicro tubes.

Apparatus

Pipet, KMP or other ultramicro type, 10 lambdas
Pipet, KMP or other ultramicro type, 100 lambdas
Pipet, KMP or other ultramicro type, 200 lambdas
Test tubes, 7 x 70 mm.
Centrifuge tubes, micro, 1 ml.

Reagents

1. *Sodium tungstate, 10 per cent:* Place 10.0 Gm. reagent quality sodium tungstate ($Na_2WO_4.2H_2O$) in a 100 ml. volumetric flask. Dissolve in distilled water and dilute to mark.

2. *Sulfuric acid, 2/3N:* Add 2.0 ml. of concentrated sulfuric acid to 116 ml. of distilled water. Mix.

3. *Precipitating reagent:* Add 5 ml. of 10 per cent sodium tungstate and 5 ml. of 2/3N H_2SO_4 to 80 ml. distilled water and mix. Store in glass stoppered reagent bottle. Discard when mixture becomes cloudy.

4. *Alkaline copper reagent (Somogyi):*

(a) Place 24 Gm. anhydrous reagent quality sodium carbonate (Na_2CO_3), 16 Gm. reagent sodium bicarbonate ($NaHCO_3$), 12 Gm. of sodium potassium tartrate ($NaKC_4H_4O_6:4H_2O$) and 90 Gm. reagent quality anhydrous sodium sulfate (Na_2SO_4) into a 500 ml. volumetric flask. Add about 400 ml. of distilled water and mix until completely dissolved. Dilute to mark with distilled water and mix.

(b) Place 4 Gm. reagent quality copper sulfate ($CuSO_4:5H_2O$) and 90 Gm. anhydrous sodium sulfate (Na_2SO_4) in a 500 ml. volumetric flask. Dissolve in about 400 ml. distilled water, dilute to mark and mix.

Mix equal parts of (a) and (b) on day of use.

5. *Phosphomolybdic acid:* Transfer to a one liter beaker 70 Gm. reagent quality molybdic acid (85 per cent MoO_3) and 10 Gm. of reagent quality sodium tungstate ($Na_2WO_4·2H_2O$). Add 400 ml. of 10 per cent sodium hydroxide solution and 400 ml. distilled water. Boil vigorously for 30-60 minutes to remove the ammonia present in the molybdic acid. Cool, dilute to about 700 ml. and add 250 ml. of 85 per cent phosphoric acid. Mix and make up to one liter volume with distilled water.

6. *Benzoic acid, 0.2 per cent:* Transfer 1 Gm. benzoic acid (C_6H_5COOH) to a 500 ml. volumetric flask, dissolve in distilled water and dilute to mark.

7. *Stock standard glucose solution:* Transfer 0.500 Gm. dry glucose to a 500 ml. volumetric flask and dilute to mark with 0.2 per cent benzoic acid. This solution keeps indefinitely.

8. *Working standard glucose solution (25 mg. per cent):* Pipet 25 ml. of stock standard glucose solution into a 100 ml. volumetric flask and dilute to mark with 0.2 per cent benzoic acid.

Procedure

1. Place 25 lambdas serum in a 1 ml. centrifuge tube.

2. Add 500 lambdas precipitating reagent and mix thoroughly by running base of tube gently back and forth over a wire test tube rack. Centrifuge for 3 minutes in a micro centrifuge.

3. Transfer 100 lambdas of clear filtrate solution to a 7 x 70 mm. test tube. Into another tube labeled *blank*, place 100 lambdas of precipitating reagent.

4. Add 100 lambdas alkaline copper reagent to each tube (prepare fresh). Mix by gentle tapping and stopper loosely. Heat in a boiling water bath for 10 minutes. Transfer to a cold water bath and cool 1-2 minutes.

5. Add 200 lambdas phosphomolybdic acid to each tube. Mix thoroughly by running base of tube gently back and forth over a wire test tube rack. When effervescence stops, add 200 lambdas distilled water and mix by inversion.

6. Read the optical density on the Beckman DU spectrophotometer. Set the instrument at 100 per cent transmittance with distilled water. Wave length 420 mμ.

Calculation

OD sample—OD blank $\times$ F = mg. per 100 ml. glucose
See calibration procedure for F.

Calibration

1. Prepare 6 glucose standard solutions by diluting 1.0, 2.0, 3.0, 4.0, 5.0 and 10.0 ml. working standard glucose solution to 10 ml. with 0.2 per cent benzoic acid and mixing well. (In this method, the diluted standards correspond to serum glucose concentrations of 52.5, 105, 157.5, 210, 262.5 and 525 mg. per 100 ml. based on a 1:21 dilution of original serum.)

2. Transfer 100 lambdas of each dilute standard to 7 x 70 mm. test tube.

3. Add 100 lambdas alkaline copper reagent to each.

4. Continue as under Procedure.

5. Calculate the factor (F) for each dilution by use of the following equation:

$$F = \frac{\text{Equivalent mg. per 100 ml. glucose}}{\text{OD } (Standard) - \text{OD } (Blank)}$$

The average value obtained is used as the factor for daily determinations.

A graph should also be plotted of optical density against equivalent serum glucose concentrations to determine adherence to Beer's law. This graph may be used for high concentrations of glucose provided at least one point is checked at the same time the test is being run.

Normal Values (Capillary or Arterial Blood)

Adults: 80-120 mg. per 100 ml. glucose in serum.

Children: 70-120 mg. per 100 ml. glucose in serum.

These values correspond to the usual Folin-Wu range. (See Discussion.) Creery and Parkinson[13] found the normal glucose range for babies 1-12 hours old to be 30-57 mg. per 100 ml. using the King-Garner method. A sharp drop was noted in the first hour after delivery. Kingsley and Getchell[23] reported that with their glucose oxidase method, normal direct plasma-glucose values of males and females from 20 and 40 years ranged between 63 and 85 mg. per 100 ml. plasma.

ENZYMATIC METHODS

Methods for the performance of glucose determinations using the specific enzyme, beta glucose oxidase, have received considerable attention since the publication of our first edition. The methods are based upon the release of hydrogen peroxide from glucose during its oxidation by glucose oxidase, conversion of the peroxide to oxygen by a peroxidase, and the detection of the oxygen by an indicator. If one of these methods is adopted for ultramicro work, it should be borne in mind that the results probably will not correspond with other procedures measuring all non-specific reducing substances in the blood; it is desirable to have the macro and the ultramicro methods similar in order to eliminate confusion if the procedures are being performed interchangeably.

Both Spinco and Coleman present ultramicro glucose oxidase methods in their manuals. Many descriptions of technics are available in the literature,[14-21] including the ultramicro method of Cawley, Spear, and Kendall[22] and that described by Kingsley and Getchell.[23] Glucose oxidase reagent is available from the Worthington Biochemical Co. (Glucostat), Takamine Laboratories, or Sigma Chemical Co. Stabilization of the color developed by the use of o-dianisidine has been recommended.[24]

ANTHRONE METHOD

A method for blood sugar estimation using anthrone has been described by Nugent and Fleming.[25] Using a blood sample of 0.05 ml., it is a composite of several methods[26-29] and is said to give reproducibility of plus or minus 5 per cent. After deproteinization with trichloroacetic acid, only one reagent is required (anthrone plus thiourea in concentrated sulfuric acid.) The handling of concentrated sulfuric acid is a disadvantage of this method; the authors recommend the use of a buret with a reservoir.

NEOCUPROINE METHOD

Ultramicro sugar determinations using 2,9-dimethyl-1,10-phenanthroline hydrochloride (Neocuproine) have been described by Brown.[32] The method replaces the phosphomolybdic acid of the Folin-Wu procedure with a solution of neocuproine; the latter is said to be thirty times more sensitive to the cuprous ion. Tests are run on the Coleman model 6A at 450 mμ.

Discussion

Determination should be carried out immediately after blood is drawn to prevent glycolysis. Capillary or arterial blood will give higher values than venous blood[1] after ingestion of glucose or food. The Somogyi alkaline copper reagent[2] is required in this ultramicro method because of the relatively large surface area of liquids contained in the micro centrifuge tubes. The final color is relatively stable and will not significantly decrease during the time required for reading in the spectrophotometer.

The ultramicro method for glucose is particularly useful for children. Children are apparently able to utilize carbohydrates to a greater degree than adults. Their renal threshold for glucose is also higher. After six years of age, a child's ability to utilize glucose gradually diminishes to that of an adult. The hyperglycemic response of children consequently varies with age as well as with body weight.

Because of the lability of blood sugar and the frequency of glycosuria in children, diagnostic errors are not uncommon. Priscilla White states that diagnosis of diabetes should be made if fasting blood sugar rises to 130 mg./100 ml., post-prandial venous blood to 170 mg./100 ml., post-prandial capillary blood sugar to 200 mg./100 ml. and if glycosuria is present.[3] Harwood uses 120 mg./100 ml. or higher as a diagnostic level for a fasting blood sugar with the post-prandial level of 200 mg./100 ml. considered as significant.[4]

Arteriovenous blood sugar differences, i.e. the divergence between blood sugars determined by the same method in venous and arterial blood, should be considered carefully. The amount of difference in the fasting state is almost negligible but after ingestion of glucose, considerable variability ensues and arterial values average somewhat higher. Mosenthal concludes from his investigations that the arterial blood furnishes more accurate information on the amount of sugar absorbed from the intestine than does venous blood, although venous blood sugar is a more accurate measure of the body's tolerance to glucose.[5]

The widely used glucose tolerance test, its modifications and its interpretations are amply covered in texts on clinical pathology and in the literature.[6-7] It need not be discussed here in great detail. Recently the concomitant use of cortisone has been introduced in order to increase the sensitivity of the test[8] and provide a possible guide for the prediction of incipient diabetes mellitus.[9] The glucose tolerance test is frequently indicated for infants and children, and ultramicro analysis is most useful.

White[3] points out that preparation for the test must be meticulous and that the patient should not receive a restricted diet, insulin or glucose for one week prior to the test. White administers 3 Gm. of glucose per Kg. of body weight to those under the age of 3 years; older patients up to the weight of 100 pounds receive 1.8 Gm. per Kg. Above 100 pounds the standard glucose tolerance test dose of 100 Gm. is administered. Blood specimens for sugar are taken fasting, one-half hour, and one-hour intervals for three hours following the single dose of glucose.

Livingston and Bridge recommended the following procedure for those under two years of age: The diet is of normal caloric value for several days and is followed by a fasting period of 12 hours for infants receiving three to five daily feedings, and 9 hours for premature infants or those receiving six or more feedings. The test dose is 3 Gm. of glucose per Kg. of body weight administered in 30 to 60 ml. of orange juice, or 1 Gm. of glucose per Kg. in a 50 per cent solution given intravenously over a period of 2-4 minutes; capillary blood is used. On a regular diet the normal blood sugar after fasting 6 to 12 hours is about 90 mg. per 100 ml.; about 70 mg. on a preceding high fat diet. A maximum blood sugar rise to 169-180 mg./100 ml. with a return to normal within 3 hours is regarded as a normal response.

Geriatric cases also require special interpretation. Chesrow and Bleyer have emphasized the importance of prolonging the oral tolerance test for at least 3 hours in patients over 60 because of the delayed return of the curve to normal.[11] Abnormal glucose tolerance tests have also been reported in patients treated with sedative drugs. The findings consisted of fasting hypoglycemia with little response to glucose, and delayed, abnormally elevated or prolonged responses.[12] These were confirmed by our own experience.

REFERENCES

1. FOSTER, G. L.: *J. Biol. Chem. 55:* 291, 1923.
2. SOMOGYI, M.: *J. Biol. Chem. 90:* 725, 1931.
3. WHITE, P.: *In* GRULLE, C. G., AND ELEY, R. C.: The Child in Health and Disease. Baltimore, Williams and Wilkins Co., 1952.
4. WHITE, P., GUEST, G. M., HARWOOD, R., AND KENNEDY, W. B.: *Diabetes 4:* 313, 1955.
5. MOSENTHAL, H. O., AND BARRY, E.: *Ann. Int. Med. 33:* 1175, 1950.
6. CONN, J. W.: *Am. J. M. Sci. 199:* 555, 1940.
7. MOYER, J. H., AND WOMACK, C. H. R.: *Am. J. M. Sci. 219:* 161, 1950.
8. BERGER, H.: *J. A. M. A. 148:* 364, 1952.
9. FAJANS, S. S., AND CONN, J. W.: *Diabetes 3:* 296, 1954.
10. LIVINGSTON, S., AND BRIDGE, E. H. M.: *J. A. M. A. 119:* 117, 1942.
11. CHESBROW, E., AND BLEYER, J. M.: *Geriatrics 9:* 276, 1954.
12. MERIVALE, W. H. H., AND HUNTER, R. A.: *Lancet 2:* 939, 1954.
13. CREERY, R. D. G., AND PARKINSON, T. J.: *Arch. Dis. Child. 28:* 134, 1953.
14. KESTON, A. S.: *Abstr. 129th Meeting Am. Chem. Soc.,* 1956, p. 31.
15. FROESCH, E. R., AND RENOLD, A. E.: *Diabetes 5:* 1, 1956.
16. TELLER, J. D.: *Abstr. 130th Meeting Am. Chem. Soc.,* 1958, p. 69.
17. MIDDLETON, J. E.: *Brit. M. J.* 824, 1959.
18. HUGGETT, A. ST. G., AND NIXON, D. A.: *Lancet 2:* 368, 1957.
19. SAIFER, A., AND GERSTENFELD, S.: *J. Lab. & Clin. Med. 51:* 448, 1958.
20. BEACH, E. F., AND TURNER, J. J.: *Clin. Chem. 4:* 462, 1958.
21. MIDDLETON, J. E.: *Brit. M. J.,* p. 824, 1959.
22. CAWLEY, L. P., SPEAR, F. E., AND KENDALL, R.: *Am. J. Clin. Path. 32:* 195, 1959.
23. KINGSLEY, G. R., AND GETCHELL, G.: *Clin. Chem. 6:* 466, 1960.
24. GUIDOTTI, G., COLOMBO, J. P., AND FOA, P. P.: *Anal. Chem. 33:* 151, 1961.
25. NUGENT, M. A., AND FLEMING, D. G.: *Am. J. Med. Tech. 24:* 8, 1958.
26. MORRIS, D.: *Science 107:* 254, 1948.
27. ZIPF, R., AND WALDO, A.: *J. Lab. & Clin. Med. 39:* 497, 1952.
28. ROE, J. H.: *J. Biol. Chem. 212:* 335, 1952.
29. HANDELSMAN, M. B., AND SASS, M.: *J. Lab. & Clin. Med. 48:* 652, 1956.
30. NELSON, N.: *J. Biol. Chem. 153:* 375, 1944.
31. SOMOGYI, M.: *J. Biol. Chem. 160:* 62, 1945.
32. BROWN, M. E.: *Diabetes 10:* 60, 1961.

12

Microhematocrits

Principle

The finger-tip or heel blood is drawn into a capillary tube which has been previously coated with anticoagulant. The bottom of this tube is sealed and the tube is spun at high speed. Speeds of centrifugation vary from 2,000 to 22,000 depending on the equipment used, but accuracy within 2 per cent can be expected when forces of 2000 g or more are used.[1]

Apparatus

No special equipment other than the ultramicro capillary tubes is actually required, but centrifuges designed particularly for microhematocrits can be purchased. The characteristics of several widely-used types are listed here. (Clay-Adams, Inc.; Drummond Scientific Co.; International Equipment Co.; Labline, Inc.)

Adams CT-2900

Capacity	24 tubes or 16 tubes in combination head
Speed	12,500 rpm
Tube size	75 mm. or smaller, including 32 mm.
Power	Electric, 115 volts, AC only; transformer available for 220 volt operation

Drummond (Figs. 39 and 40)

Capacity	16 tubes
Speed	16,500 rpm
Tube size	32 mm. x 0.8 mm. O.D.
Power	Electric, 115 volts, AC or DC

Labline Model 31 (Fig. 42)

Capacity	36 or 16 tubes in combination head
Speed	12,000 rpm

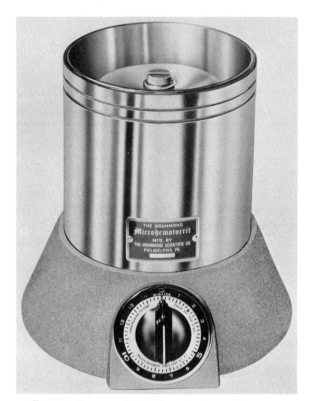

Fig. 39.—Drummond microhematocrit centrifuge.

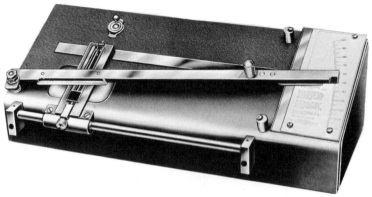

Fig. 40.—Drummond hematocrit reader.

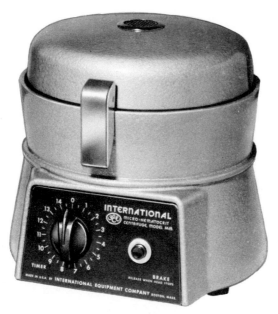

Fig. 41.—International hematocrit centrifuge.

Labline Model 31 (Cont.)

Tube size   75 x 1.75 mm.; 75 x 7 mm.
Power   Electric, 115 volts, AC or DC

International Model MB (Fig. 44)

Capacity   24 tubes or 16 tubes in combination head
Speed   11,500 to 15,000 (depending on head used)
Tube size   75 x 1.5 mm. up to 73 x 7 mm.
Power   Electric, 115 volts, AC. 230 volt model
                          available at extra cost

Where only a few hematocrits are run, the Adams micro-chemistry centrifuge, CT-3000, is adaptable to micro-hematocrit determinations by interchanging the 8-place micro-chemistry head with a 16-place or 24-place micro-hematocrit head. Similarly, the International clinical centrifuge may be adapted by use of their "Hematokit," providing a capacity of 24 75 x 1.5 mm. tubes at a speed of 7500 rpm (Fig. 43). Heads for spinning 1 ml. micro centrifuge tubes are available for both the clinical and microcapillary International models (Figs. 43, 44). Busier laboratories will require separate centrifuges.

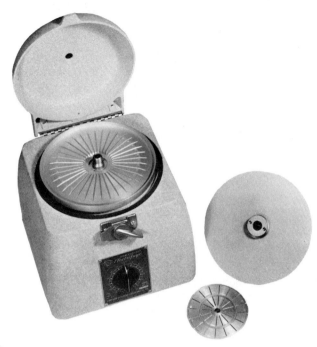

Fig. 42.—Chicago Surgical Electric Co., Div. of Labline, Inc., hematocrit centrifuge with interchangeable heads.

All of the above centrifuges should prove satisfactory, but before making a choice it is advisable to *hear* a centrifuge as well as see it, as some models are considerably quieter than others. Sound-muffling boxes may be constructed, but one should be careful not to overheat the centrifuge.

Reagents

Anticoagulants that may be used include saturated ammonium oxalate, ammonium citrate, double oxalate or heparin. The ammonium oxalate is approximately 2.5 per cent solution. The ammonium citrate is prepared by dissolving 3 Gm. of citric acid dihydrate in 50 ml. water and adding concentrated ammonium hydroxide until neutral to litmus.[2] The 1 per cent double oxalate solution is prepared according to Strumia[3] by dissolving 0.6 Gm. of ammonium oxalate monohydrate and 0.4 Gm. of potassium oxalate monohydrate in distilled water, diluting to 100 ml. and mixing. Heparin must be diluted 3 mg./ml. and allowed to dry on the inner surfaces of the tubes prior to use. Heparinized or oxalated capillary tubes may be obtained from commercial sources.

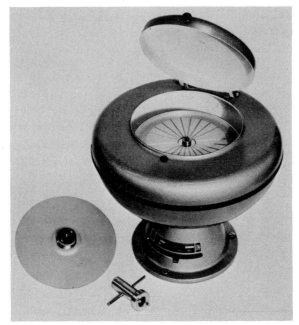

Fig. 43.—International clinical centrifuge model 428, with Hematokit 930.

Procedure

1. Take blood from the finger or heel directly into a heparinized or oxalated capillary tube. The blood should flow freely—avoid squeezing the tissue!

2. The tube may be sealed over a hot gas flame; larger tubes must be rotated to provide a flat bottom. If the regular ultramicro collection tube is used, the end may be sealed with cement or wax and the capillary tube then placed in a macro test tube. Sealing materials are also available commercially. (Seal-Ease, Clay-Adams, Inc.; Critoseal, Biological Research, Inc.) Seal-Ease is a clay containing numbered double trough and Critoseal has 36 numbered openings over a uniform layer of vinyl plastic putty.

3. Prepare a list of patients' names, noting the numbers assigned in the centrifuge.

4. Centrifuge specimens three to two minutes in a high speed centrifuge (11,000-16,000 rpm) or 30 minutes at 2000 rpm.

5. Measure with calipers and a centimeter rule, or use commercial reading aids. (Clay-Adams, Inc.; Drummond Scientific Co.; Labline, Inc.; International Equipment Co.)

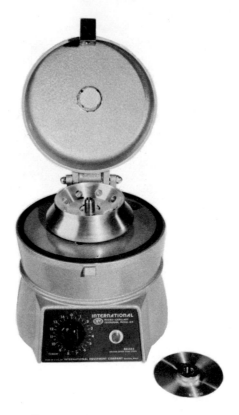

Fig. 44.—Micro-capillary centrifuge, model MB, International Equipment Co.

Normal Values

Thanks to the investigations of DeMarsh et al.[4-6] we are now able to interpret some of the wide variations found in the blood picture at birth. The time at which the umbilical cord was clamped, the time after birth at which the sample was obtained and the site from which the blood is taken all influence the findings. On blood taken from the superior saggital sinus, mean hematocrit values were reported as follows:[6]

	Umbilical cord clamped immediately	Cords clamped after placental separation
First day	52 per cent	60 per cent
Third day	50 per cent	59 per cent

Similar results were also obtained from blood drawn from the heel. The

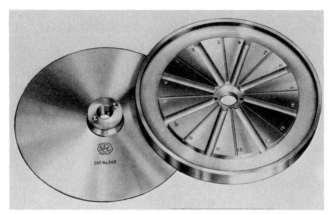

Fig. 45.—Combination head for micro-capillary centrifuge, model MB, International Equipment Co.

heel blood showed a significantly higher hemoglobin and erythrocyte count, but no significant difference in the hematocrit.[6, 8]

Kolmer[9] lists the following normal values for packed erythrocytes per 100 ml. of blood:

Infants..49 to 60 ml.
Children...35 to 44 ml.
Men..41 to 52 ml.
Women..38 to 46 ml.

Strumia's figures are given on p. 116.

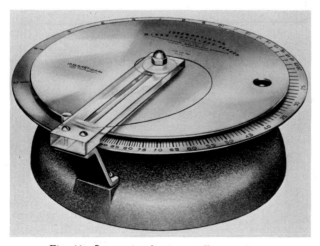

Fig. 46.—International microcapillary reader.

When accurately measured, 1 hematocrit unit is equal approximately to 0.34 Gm. of hemoglobin per 100 mm., or 107,000 erythrocytes per cu. mm., provided the cells are normochromic and normocytic.[47]

TABLE 4.—CHILDREN OF BOTH SEXES

Age	Average Normal	Minimum Normal
Birth	56.6	51.0
First Day	56.1	50.5
End of 1st wk.	52.7	47.5
End of 2nd wk.	49.6	44.7
End of 3rd wk.	46.6	42.0
End of 4th wk.	44.6	40.0
End of 2nd mo.	38.9	35.1
End of 4th mo.	36.5	32.9
End of 6th mo.	36.2	32.6
End of 1st yr.	35.2	31.7
End of 2nd yr.	35.5	32.0
End of 4th yr.	37.1	33.4
End of 6th yr.	37.9	34.2
End of 8th yr.	38.9	35.1
End of 12th yr.	39.6	35.7

TABLE 5.—HEMOGLOBIN-HEMATOCRIT-ERYTHROCYTE COUNT

Hemoglobin	Hematocrit	Erythrocyte
10.20	30	3.210000
10.54	31	3.317000
10.88	32	3.424000
11.22	33	3.531000
11.56	34	3.638000
11.90	35	3.745000
12.24	36	3.852000
12.58	37	3.959000
12.92	38	4.066000
13.26	39	4.173000
13.60	40	4.280000
13.94	41	4.387000
14.28	42	4.494000
14.62	43	4.601000
14.96	44	4.708000
15.30	45	4.815000
15.64	46	4.922000
15.98	47	5.029000
16.32	48	5.136000
16.66	49	5.243000
17.00	50	5.350000

Reproduced by permission, from data compiled by Dr. Max Strumia.

Discussion

According to Wintrobe,[10] the hematocrit was introduced in the latter part of the Nineteenth Century. It has had slow acceptance and its worth has been bitterly contested. However, it is at last assuming its rightful place as one of the most valuable examinations in our hematologic armamentarium. Wintrobe's own hematocrit tube, requiring one ml. of blood, is widely used. But there is also growing interest in other methods, many of which utilize smaller quantities of capillary blood. Van Allen, Mason, Kaldor, Guest and Siler, Strumia and many others have presented methods and variations of hematocrit determination.[2, 11-34] These vary from the extremely simple to the highly complex; "from the sublime to the ridiculous."

The test itself is fundamentally simple. Non-coagulated blood is centrifuged and the volume of packed erythrocytes is compared with the total volume and a percentage is derived. The controversies have arisen over the surface area of the fluid, the amount of plasma "trapped" among the erythrocytes and the effects of the container wall. The mathematical gyrations, claims and counter-claims have resulted in so much contention that the fundamental value of the test has often been overshadowed.[1, 35-45]

Unfortunately, the *statistically* significant differences which undoubtedly occur have been used interchangeably with *clinically* significant differences, which is not always synonomous. Coefficients of variation of 1.3 per cent are hardly worrisome from a clinical standpoint. And we are inclined to agree with McGovern et al.[33] that the microhematocrit method is dependable and gives highly reproducible results and that capillary blood methods give satisfactory results.

An electronic method of measuring hematocrits has been made available.[48] Utilizing the principle that the electrical resistance of a column of blood is a function of the relative volume per 100 ml. of erythrocytes, this method is performed in a transistorized portable unit powered by a radio battery.* The small sample size (0.02 ml.) permits measurements on ultramicro quantities and a reading is provided within 30 seconds. Only heparinized or whole blood have been found satisfactory in this instrument; oxalate is said to alter the conductivity. We have not personally evaluated this electronic micro-hematocrit method.

One ml. of whole blood is required to raise the hematocrit value of the patient's blood one unit per pound of body weight.[46] Thus, if a premature baby weighs 4 pounds, with an hematocrit of 35 per cent, a 40 per cent rise requires: 1 x 5 x 4—20 ml. whole blood.

---

* YSI Model 30 electronic micro-hematocrit, Scientific Products Div., Am. Hospital Supply Corp.

REFERENCES

1. VAZQUEZ, O. N., NEWERLY, K., YALOW, R., AND BERSON, S. A.: *J. Lab. & Clin. Med.* *39:* 595, 1952.
2. NATELSON, S.: *Am. J. Clin. Path. 21:* 1153, 1951.
3. STRUMIA, M. M., SAMPLE, A. B., AND HART, E. D.: *Am. J. Clin. Path. 24:* 1016, 1954.
4. DE MARSH, Q. B., WINDLE, W. F., AND ALT, H. L.: *Am J. Dis. Child. 63:* 1123, 1942.
5. —————, ALT, H. L., WINDLE, W. F., AND HILLIS, D. S.: *J. A. M. A. 116:* 2563, 1941.
6. —————, —————, AND —————: *Am. J. Dis. Child. 75:* 860, 1948.
7. SMITH, C. A.: The Physiology of the Newborn. Springfield, Ill., C. C Thomas, 1945.
8. HADEN, R. L., AND NEFF, F. C.: *Am. J. Dis. Child. 28:* 458, 1924.
9. KOLMER, J. A., SPAULDING, E. H., AND ROBINSON H.: Approved Laboratory Technic. New York Appleton-Century-Crofts, 1951.
10. WINTROBE, M. M.: Clinical Hematology. Philadelphia, Lea & Febiger, 1951.
11. EPSTEIN, A. A.: *J. Lab. Clin. Med. 1:* 610, 1915.
12. CAMPBELL, J. M. H.: *Brit. J. Exper. Path. 3:* 217, 1922.
13. HADEN, R. L.: *Arch. Int. Med. 31:* 766, 1923.
14. VAN ALLEN, C. M.: *J.A.M.A. 84:* 202, 1925.
15. —————: *J. Lab. Clin. Med. 10:* 1027, 1925.
16. SMIRK, F. H.: *Brit. J. Exper. Path. 9:* 81, 1928.
17. SANFORD, A. H., AND MAGATH, T. B.: *J. Lab. & Clin. Med. 15:* 172, 1929.
18. HADEN, R. L.: *J. Lab. & Clin. Med. 15:* 736, 1930.
19. PONDER, E., AND SASLOW, G.: *J. Physiol. 70:* 18, 1930.
20. HADEN, R. L.: *Am. J. M. Sc. 181:* 597, 1931.
21. OSGOOD, E. E., HASKINS, H. D., AND TROTMAN, F. E.: *J. Lab. & Clin. Med. 16:* 476, 1931.
22. ROSAHN, P. D.: *Proc. Soc. Exper. Biol. & Med. 28:* 491, 1931.
23. HADEN, R. L.: *J. Lab. & Clin. Med. 17:* 843, 1932.
24. SLAWINSKI, A.: *Biochem. J. 27:* 356, 1933.
25. MASON, S. J.: *J. Lab. & Clin. Med. 20:* 318, 1934.
26. GUEST, G. M., AND SILER, V. E.: *J. Lab. & Clin. Med. 19:* 757, 1934.
27. MILLER, A. T., JR.: *J. Lab. & Clin. Med. 24:* 547, 1939.
28. HAMRE, C. J.: *J. Lab. & Clin. Med. 25:* 547, 1940.
29. MEYERSTEIN, W.: *J. Physiol. 101:* 5, 1942.
30. SMITH, S. E.: *J. Lab. & Clin. Med. 29:* 301, 1944.
31. STRUMIA, M.: *Am. J. Clin. Path. 20:* 1180, 1948.
32. KALDOR, I.: *Med. J. Aus. 13:* 476, 1953.
33. McGOVERN, J. J., JONES, A. R., AND STEINBERG, A. G.: New England *J. Med. 253:* 308, 1955.
34. JONES, A. R.: New England *J. Med. 254:* 172, 1956.
35. HIROTA, K.: *J. Biophys. 1:* 233, 1925.
36. MILLAR, D. G.: *Quart. J. Exper. Physiol. 15:* 187, 1925.
37. PONDER, E., AND SASLOW, G.: *J. Physiol. 70:* 18, 1930.
38. WINTROBE, M. M.: *Am. J. Clin. Path. 1:* 147, 1931.
39. CHAPIN, M. A., AND ROSS, J. F.: *Am. J. Physiol. 137:* 447, 1942.
40. MAIZELS, M.: *Quart. J. Exper. Physiol. 33:* 129, 1945.
41. MAYERSON, H. A., LYONS, C., PARSONS, W., NEISET, T., AND TRAUTMAN, W.: *Am. J. Physiol. 155:* 232, 1948.
42. BARNES, D. W. H., LOUITT, J. F., AND REEVE, E. B.: *Clin. Sc. 7:* 135, 1948.

43. PONDER, E.: Hemolysis and Related Phenomena, New York, Grune & Stratton, 1948.
44. JACKSON, M. D., AND NUTT, M. E.: *J. Physiol. 115:* 196, 1951.
45. LIESON, D., AND REEVE, E. B.: *J. Physiol. 115:* 129, 1951.
46. NATELSON, S., CRAWFORD, W. L., AND MUNSEY, F. A.: Correlation of Clinical and Chemical Observations in the Immature Infant. Richmond Hill, Endo Products, New York, 1952.
47. WOLMAN, I. J.: Laboratory Applications in Clinical Pediatrics. New York, McGraw-Hill, 1957.
48. KERNEN, J. A., WURZEL, H., AND OKADA, R.: *J. Lab. & Clin. Med. 57:* 635, 1961.

13

Icterus Index

Principle

The intensity of the yellow color of serum is compared with a standard potassium dichromate solution and the results expressed in units.[1,2] This color at the wavelength used in this procedure will primarily represent the bilirubin level. This ultramicro procedure may be calibrated by using serum samples previously analyzed in duplicate with a standard macro method or by the direct use of potassium dichromate. The wavelength and potassium dichromate concentration used here were suggested by Henry.[2]

Apparatus

Pipet, KMP or other ultramicro type, 10 lambdas
Pipet, KMP or other ultramicro type, 200 lambdas
Test tubes, 7 x 70 mm.

Reagents

1. *Sodium citrate, 5.0 per cent:* Transfer 5.0 Gm. sodium citrate to a 100 ml. volumetric flask, dissolve in distilled water and dilute to mark. Add a few drops of chloroform as a preservative.

2. *Stock potassium dichromate standard solution:* Transfer 1.57 Gm. reagent quality potassium dichromate, $K_2Cr_2O_7$, to a 100 ml. volumetric flask. Dissolve in about 70 ml. distilled water, add 1 drop of concentrated sulfuric acid, dilute to mark and mix. Store in glass-stoppered brown bottle.

Procedure

1. **Pipet 10 lambdas of serum into a 7 x 70 mm. test tube.**
2. **Add 200 lambdas 5 per cent sodium citrate solution and mix by gentle tapping.**

3. Read the optical density of this mixture in a Beckman DU or other spectrophotometer at 460 mμ^2 using distilled water to set the instrument at 100 per cent transmittance.

Calculations

Optical density $\times$ F = icterus index in units
See *Calibration* for Factor (F)

Calibration

1. Obtain several samples of clear unhemolyzed serum with varying degrees of icterus. Determine the icterus index on each sample by a standard macro procedure.

2. Using the same specimens, analyze as given above under procedure. Calculate a conversion factor as follows:

$$F = \frac{\text{icterus index (macro)}}{\text{OD (micro)}}$$

Or:

1. Dilute 0.5, 1.0, 2.0, 3.0 and 5.0 ml. of stock potassium dichromate standard solution to 100 ml. with distilled water. These standards correspond to an icterus index of 10.5, 21, 42 and 105 units based on a 1:21 dilution of the original serum.

2. Dilute and read as given above under *Procedure.*

$$F = \frac{\text{equivalent icterus index}}{\text{OD (standard)}}$$

The mean of the F values for each standard may be determined and used as a factor. A calibration curve should be prepared to determine the extent of the linearity of the curve.

Normal Values

3-8 units

Discussion

When this method is calibrated against a similar macro method, the values obtained from both technics will agree. This is a more satisfactory procedure since the icterus index units are arbitrary and will vary between different spectrophotometers and technics. Blood should be obtained in a fasting state to avoid lipemia. The icterus index is not an accurate laboratory test, but it is simple and will often serve a useful purpose. It is difficult to compare with the bilirubin level, although it tends to run eight to ten times as high as the number of mg. of bilirubin per 100 cc.[3]

The icterus index may rise to 15 units without clinical signs of jaundice. It will be elevated in diseases of the liver or bile tract and in extrahepatic hemolytic disorders such as erythroblastosis. Birth injuries with resultant hemorrhage may cause a moderate elevation of serum bilirubin and the icterus index.

Infants who are apparently normal are frequently jaundiced after the third day of life; the icterus disappears by the tenth day. This is called "physiologic jaundice" and seems to be the result of erythrocyte destruction plus transient functional inadequacy of the liver. It reaches higher levels and persists considerably longer in the premature infant.[4] Icterus appearing within the first 12 hours of life usually indicates erythroblastosis fetalis.[5] Because of its rapid progression and difficult prognosis it is often called "icterus gravis."

REFERENCES

1. MEULENGRACHT, E. D.: *Arch. klin. Med. 132:* 285, 1920.
2. HENRY, R. J., GOLUB, O. J., BERKMAN, S., AND SEGALOVE, M.: *Am. J. Clin. Path. 23:* 841, 1953.
3. HOFFMAN, W. S.: The Biochemistry of Clinical Medicine, Ed. 2, Chicago, Year Book Publ., Inc., 1959.
4. WOLMAN, I. J.: Laboratory Applications in Clinical Pediatrics. New York, McGraw-Hill, 1957.
5. POTTER, E. L.: Pathology of the Fetus and the Newborn. Chicago, Year Book Publ., Inc., 1952.

14

Microflocculation Tests for Syphilis

Some of the serologic tests for syphilis have been designed or modified to provide procedures which may be used when only small amounts of plasma or serum are available. As this situation usually exists in patients where ultramicro chemistry is indicated, representative methods are included. Those selected are the plasmacrit,[1] the Davies-Hinton, and the Mazzini microflocculation tests. The latter two are performed on serum. A Kahn microflocculation test using cardiolipin antigen is also available.

The results of these serologic tests are accurate only when the author's technics are carefully followed and the tests are performed with standardized reagents and *known positive controls*. Each new batch of reagent should be compared with that already in use before being accepted for routine utilization.

PLASMACRIT (PCT) TEST OF ANDUJAR AND MAZUREK

This test was developed by Andujar and Mazurek[1] to utilize the unheated waste plasma from microhematocrit capillary tubes. Plasma is known to be superior to serum for serologic tests for syphilis because of its high reagin content. Inactivation is performed chemically instead of by heat; choline chloride gives satisfactory specificity and good sensitivity in the screening test. The procedure can be performed in only a few minutes. The sensitivity of the plasmacrit test is greater than Kahn, Kline, or VDRL tests. Harris, Sunkes, Bunch, and Bossak[2] did a comparative study with the PCT and slide VDRL on 708 specimens, with greater correlation of the PCT in the group with higher probability of past or present syphilitic infection. The test is considered highly sensitive, reasonably specific, reasonably simple, inexpensive, and free of danger of serum hepatitis.[3] These factors, plus its rapid performance, appear to make it an excellent screening flocculation test. It should not be regarded as diagnostic, and all positives should be followed up with standard serologic tests.

Apparatus

Microhematocrit centrifuge
Rotating machine, Kline or VDRL type, 180 rpm, circle ¾" in diameter
Heparinized capillary plasmacrit (PCT) tubes. *Note:* Ordinary micro-
hematocrit tubes are not satisfactory.
Sealing material (Critoseal, Scientific Products)
VDRL slide antigen and VDRL saline
Choline chloride (Eastman Kodak #1122)
Serologic ceramic ring test plates
Tuberculin syringe, 2 ml. size, with 25 gauge needle with bevel removed,
calibrated to deliver 100 drops/ml.
Small vaccine bulbs (Scientific Products #52215)
Centrifuge capable of centrifugal force of 2000 g

Reagents

Antigen emulsion
Choline chloride mixture
(See specific instruction by Andujar and Mazurek[1])

Preparing Reagents

Choline chloride—A solution of 10 ml. of 10 per cent choline chloride in
0.85 per cent saline should be made when the emulsion is to be prepared.
It should be refrigerated.

Antigen emulsion—VDRL slide emulsion is prepared as specified in *Serologic Tests for Syphilis*,[4] but after the 5 ml. of the antigen emulsion is ready
it is centrifuged in a conical stainless steel tube in an angle centrifuge at
approximately 2000 g for 15-30 minutes. The supernatant fluid is discarded
and the emulsion of antigen is resuspended by blowing 5 ml. of 10 per cent
choline chloride in saline directly onto the sediment and then vigorously
agitating the centrifuge tube. This is to rid the emulsion of traces of alcohol
which might interfere with the antiinhibitor effect of the choline chloride.
The emulsion may be kept several weeks in the refrigerator, but aliquots
should be warmed to room temperature prior to use.

Procedure

1. After the usual cleaning with alcohol, the fingertip is pierced

deeply with a sterile, disposable lancet, in order to obtain a free flow of capillary blood.

2. The special PCT capillary tube is filled to within 5 to 10 mm. of the free end, and then gently rotated or tilted (with both ends open) in order to mix the blood and heparin preparation.

3. The dry end of the tube is plugged with Critoseal, and then the blood is centrifuged in a microhematocrit centrifuge for approximately 3 minutes at 11,000 rpm. If desired, the volume of packed red blood cells may be observed at this time.

4. From the free end of the column of plasma, a length of 22 mm. (no less than 22 mm. and no more than 26 m.) is marked toward the packed red blood cells, the capillary tube is broken at this point and, by means of a small rubber bulb fitted to the tube, the plasma is expelled onto a ring-plate.

5. One drop (0.01 ml.) of antigen emulsion (previously treated with choline chloride as an anti-inhibitor) is added to the 0.023 to 0.020 ml. of plasma, and the mixture is agitated on a serologic rotator for 4 minutes and then promptly observed for clumping. Adequate control tests with known reactive plasma should always be included.

Interpretation

On the basis of the amount of microscopic flocculation observed, the results of the PCT test are reported in the following manner:

1. No clumping—"nonreactive or negative."
2. Only slight clumping—"weakly reactive or doubtful." (The test should be repeated with another specimen.)
3. Moderate to conspicuous clumping—"reactive" (submit serum).

In the third category, the requested specimen of serum should be studied by means of various standard serologic tests for syphilis.

DAVIES-HINTON MICROFLOCCULATION TEST WITH SERUM

Reagents

Rubber caps (#3 vial stoppers).
Glass tubing, approximately 80 x 2.5 mm. bore.
Capillary pipet, 10 x 1 cm. diameter (capillary end approximately 1 mm. in diameter).

Apparatus

1. *Hinton indicator:* An alcoholic solution containing 0.0884 per cent cardiolipin, 0.6188 per cent purified lecithin and 0.24 per cent cholesterol. Each lot of antigen is serologically standardized by proper comparison with an antigen of known reactivity.

2. *Sodium chloride solution, five per cent:* Weigh 5 Gm. of previously dried sodium chloride (A.C.S.). Add sodium chloride to 100 ml. of distilled water and heat solution in an autoclave at 15 lbs. pressure for 15 minutes. Store saline solution in a glass stoppered bottle at room temperature (73 to 85 F.).

3. *Sodium chloride solution, 0.85 per cent:* Add 8.5 Gm. dried sodium chloride to liter of distilled water. This solution should be prepared on the day used.

4. *Glycerin solution, fifty per cent:* Mix equal volumes of Baker and Adamson's glycerin (reagent grade) and distilled water. This solution keeps indefinitely. (Allied Chemical and Dye Corp.)

Preparing Glycerinated Hinton Indicator

1. Pipet one part Hinton stock indicator into one compartment of a Hinton flask. Mix not less than 1 ml. nor more than 5 ml. of Hinton indicator at a time.

2. Pipet 0.8 part of 5 per cent sodium chloride solution into the other compartment of the flask. Use care in pipetting the solution to avoid *premature mixing* of the solutions.

3. Mix contents by shaking flask rapidly for one minute and let mixture stand *exactly 5 minutes.*

4. Add 13.2 parts of 5 per cent sodium chloride solution and shake flask vigorously.

5. Add 15 parts of 50 per cent glycerine solution and shake until the suspension is homogeneous.

6. Store in a glass-stoppered bottle or flask under refrigeration. This suspension remains usable for at least three weeks.

Preparing Serums

1. Collect capillary blood in the usual manner.[5] The cap is then removed and a wire may be used to loosen the clot from the side of the tube if necessary.

2. Place capped collecting tube in a labeled test tube and centrifuge at high speed for 10 minutes, or until serum is well separated from clot.

3. Add water to the test tubes containing the capped blood collecting tubes and place in a 56 C. water bath for 30 minutes.

4. Remove tubes from water bath and discard water from the test tubes; then remove cap from the serum end of the collection tube, notch and break just above the junction of clot and serum. Discard the portion of the tube containing the clot.

Procedure

1. **Transfer each serum to two glass collection tubes. One tube should contain a column of serum about 2.5 cm. high and the other a column 0.5 to 1.0 cm. high.**
2. **Add to the tube containing the higher (2.5 cm.) column an equal amount of glycerinated Hinton indicator. Use the capillary pipet for the indicator. Be sure indicator comes into *direct contact* with serum.**
3. **Add a column of 2.5 cm. to 5.0 cm. in length of glycerinated Hinton indicator to the serum in the second tube (0.5 to 1.0 cm. column).**
4. **Mix the serum and glycerinated Hinton indicator in each tube by tilting the liquid toward alternate ends of the tube *10 times*.**
5. **Cap both ends of the tube collection tubes and place them in test tubes that are identically numbered.**
6. **Fill the test tubes containing capped collection tubes with water and place in 37 C. water bath for *16 hours*.**
7. **Remove tubes from water bath, pour water from test tubes, and centrifuge the tubes containing capped collection tubes five minutes at *approximately 2000 rpm*.**

Reading Test Results

The results are read under the low power objective of microscope under reduced light. The microscope stage should be tilted approximately 30° from horizontal and the tube placed under the lens with a meniscus uppermost. Observe if any clumping is present at the meniscus and report as follows:

Reactive: Definite discrete compact clumps at the meniscus in either tube. (*Positive.*) Gentle tapping of tube may help float clumps into view.

Non-reactive: No clumps visible in either tube. (*Negative.*) Amorphous, cloudy, granular particles at the meniscus are also interpreted as non-reactive or "negative."

Weakly reactive: Small clumps at the meniscus of either tube. (*Doubtful.*) In such instances, clumps should be redispersed by tapping the tube with a finger, again centrifuging tube for 3 minutes. The test is reported as weakly reactive or "doubtful" if small clumps are again visible at the meniscus; but is reported reactive or "positive" if large compact clumps are present in either tube.

MAZZINI MICROFLOCCULATION TEST WITH SERUM

Apparatus

Rubber caps (#3 vial stoppers)
Glass tubing, 80 mm. x 2.5 mm. bore
Rotating machine, 100-180 rpm circle ¾ inch in diameter
Slide holder for several 2 x 3 inch slides
Hypodermic needles, 13 and 21 gauge, bevels removed
Glass slides, 2 x 3 inches with 10 concavities 16 mm. wide by 3 mm. deep
Syringe, 1 or 2 ml. capacity

It is also possible to use glass slides 2 x 3 inches with 15 mm. paraffin or ceramic rings. Ring making machines are commercially available.

Reagents

1. *Mazzini cholesterolized antigen:* Available commercially. (Sylvana Chemical Corp.)

2. *Buffered 1 per cent saline solution, pH 6.3 to 6.4:* Available commercially. (Sylvana Chemical Corp.)

Preparing Antigen Emulsion

1. Pipet 0.4 ml. of buffered saline solution to the bottom of a small bottle.

2. Measure 0.4 ml. of cholesterolized antigen with a 1 ml. pipet graduated to the tip.

3. While the saline solution is being rotated in the hand, add the antigen *quickly* into the solution.

4. Mix by drawing the suspension into the pipet and blowing out six times. Be careful to empty the pipet *completely* into the final mixture.

5. Add 2.6 ml. of the buffered saline solution, cap the bottle and shake from bottom to top 50 times in 15 seconds. Allow this suspension to stand at room temperature for 3 hours. It is then usable for the following 5 hours.

6. Emulsion is now ready for immediate use and remains usable for 8 hours. It should be shaken gently each time prior to use.

7. Transfer suspension to a 5 ml. syringe fitted with a 25 gauge needle.

Preparing Serums

1. Collect capillary blood in the usual manner.[5]

2. Place the capped collecting tube in a labeled test tube and centrifuge at high speed for 10 minutes or until serum is well separated from clot.

3. Add water to the test tubes containing the capped blood collecting tubes and place in a 56 C. water bath for 30 minutes. Sera should be reheated

for 10 minutes if re-examined more than 4 hours after the original heating period.

4. Recentrifuge any specimen in which visible particles have formed during heating.

5. Remove the cap from the serum end of the collecting tube, file and break tube just above the junction of the serum clot. Discard the clot-filled portion of the tube.

Preliminary Tests

Check delivery of the syringe that is fitted with a 21 gauge needle so it will deliver 0.01 ml. of antigen per drop.

Test the control sera of graded reactivity and the buffered saline solution. The reactivity pattern previously established for these sera should be reproduced and should show complete dispersion of the antigen particles in both non-reactive (negative) and buffered saline solutions.

Procedure

1. Pipet 0.03 ml. of each serum into a separate concavity.
2. Add 1 drop of antigen emulsion (0.01 ml.) to each serum.
3. Rotate slides on machine *for 4 minutes*. The speed should be 160 to 180 rotations per minute. (Rotation may be done by circumscribing a 2-inch circle 120 times per minute.)
4. Read each reaction microscopically under the low power objective and a 5X ocular. Record and report all sera that are non-reactive or *negative* and all serums that are reactive or *positive*.
5. Add 1 drop (about 0.05 ml.) of 0.9 per cent saline solution from a syringe, using a 13 gauge needle with bevel removed, to each test giving a 1, 2, 3 plus, or atypical reaction.
6. Rotate the slide for *another* 4-minute period on rotating machine set at 100-120 rpm or by hand.
7. Examine under the microscope. Results are reported as follows:

Typical Reactions

Description	Reading	Report
No clumping	Negative	Non-reactive—negative
Very small clumps	1+	Weakly reactive—doubtful
Small clumps	2+	Reactive—positive
Medium size clumps	3+	Reactive—positive
Large clumps	4+	Reactive—positive

Atypical Reactions

These are characterized by irregular aggregations of particles of various sizes in which the small clumps of free antigen particles predominate. They should be retested using the Mazzini quantitative test and other serologic testing methods.

Discussion

The serologic tests described above are nonspecific indications of syphilitic infections. While useful as screening procedures, they should be supplemented in questionable cases by other tests based on test tube agglutination, complement fixation or *Treponema pallidum* immobilization. Like biochemical determinations, serologic tests have undergone continual modification[9-11] and considerable improvements can be expected in the future. Syphilis can be diagnosed only by the physician who examines the patient and *not* by a laboratory test.

REFERENCES

1. ANDUJAR, J. J., AND MAZUREK, E. E.: *Am. J. Clin. Path. 31:* 197, 1959.
2. HARRIS, A., SUNKES, E. J., BUNCH, W. L., AND BOSSAK, H. N.: *Pub. Health Lab. 17:* 83, 1959.
3. CAWLEY, L.: Personal communication.
4. U. S. DEPARTMENT OF HEALTH, EDUCATION AND WELFARE: Serological Tests for Syphilis. Washington, 1955.
5. DAVIES, J. A. V.: *J. Lab. & Clin. Med. 23:* 1206-1209, 1938.
6. STUART, G. O., GRANT, J. F., AND HINTON, W. A.: *J. Ven. Dis. Inform. 29:* 27, 1948.
7. HINTON, W. A., STUART, G. O., AND GRANT J. F.: *Am. J. Syph. 33:* 587-592, 1959.
8. MAZZINI, L. Y.: *J. Immunol. 66:* 261-276, 1951.
9. GARSON, W.: *Ann. Int. Med. 51:* 748, 1959.
10. REIN, C. R., AND KELCEC, L. C.: *J.A.M.A. 163:* 1046, 1957.
11. PATTON, R. B., AND GAURIE, A. : *Am. J. Clin. Path. 36:* 383, 1961.

15

Non-Protein Nitrogen

Principle

A protein-free filtrate of the serum is prepared by the tungstic acid procedure. Organic compounds present in the protein-free filtrate are oxidized with H_2SO_4 and hydrogen peroxide. Nitrogen present in these compounds is converted to NH_3. The solution is diluted and Nessler's reagent added, developing color in proportion to the amount of ammonium ion. Photometric comparison is made with a solution containing a known amount of nitrogen in the form of ammonium ion.[1]

Apparatus

Pipets, KMP or other ultramicro type, 25 lambdas
Pipets, KMP or other ultramicro type, 100 lambdas
Pipets, KMP or other ultramicro types, 200 lambdas or 400 lambdas
Pipet, KMP or other ultramicro type, 250 lambdas
Pyrex test tube, graduated at 2 ml.
Microburner
Glass beads

Reagents

1. *Sulfuric acid, 1:1 dilution:* Dilute one volume concentrated sulfuric acid with an equal volume distilled water. Cool and store in a glass-stoppered bottle.

2. *Hydrogen peroxide solution, 30 per cent:* This must be nitrogen-free. Satisfactory preparations are available on the market, such as Merck's or Baker's. Hydrogen peroxide deteriorates in storage and should be vented to avoid developing excessive internal pressure. Store in a cool place and protect from light.

3. *Gum-ghatti solution:* Fill a one-liter graduated cylinder to the one-liter mark with distilled water. Just below the surface suspend 20 Gm. of soluble

gum-ghatti by means of a cloth bag. Allow to stand overnight or longer. Remove the undissolved material and filter the solution through coarse filter paper.

4. *Koch-McMeekin Nessler solution:* We recommend the use of commercially available solution. If desired, prepare as follows:

Dissolve 30 Gm. of potassium iodide in 20 ml. of distilled water and add 22.5 Gm. iodine to the solution. Shake until dissolved and add 30 Gm. pure metallic mercury.

Shake the mixture well, keeping the solution cool by holding under running tap water until the supernatant liquid has lost the yellow color of iodine.

Pour off from the undissolved mercury and test for the presence of excess iodine by adding a few drops of the clear solution to 1 ml. of a 1 per cent starch solution in a test tube. If there is no blue color, add iodine solution similar to that described above, drop by drop, until there is a faint excess of free iodine. Dilute to 200 ml. and pour into 975 ml. of 10 per cent sodium hydroxide solution. Mix well and allow any precipitate to settle out. Use the clear supernatant fluid. Avoid stirring.

5. *Protein precipitating reagent:*

a. *Sodium tungstate, 10 per cent:*   Place 10.0 Gm. reagent quality sodium tungstate ($Na_2Wo_4 \cdot H_2O$) in a 100 ml. volumetric flask. Dissolve in distilled water and dilute to mark.

b. *Sulfuric acid, 2/3 N:*   Add 2.0 ml. concentrated sulfuric acid to 116 ml. of distilled water. Mix.

c. *Protein-precipitating reagent:*   Add 5 ml. of 10 per cent sodium tungstate and 5 ml. of 2/3N H_2SO_4 to 80 ml. distilled water and mix. Store in glass-stoppered bottle. Discard mixture when it becomes cloudy.

Procedure

1.   Pipet 25 lambdas of serum into a 1 ml. centrifuge tube.

2.   Add 500 lambdas of protein-precipitating reagent and mix thoroughly. Centrifuge for 3 minutes in a micro centrifuge.

3.   Transfer 250 lambdas of the protein-free supernatant into a pyrex test tube graduated at 2 ml.

4.   Add 25 lambdas of diluted sulfuric acid.

5.   Add one small clean glass bead.

Heat over a micro burner until the water has been driven off and dense white fumes fill the tube. With the tube in an upright position, drop directly into the solution one drop of 30 per cent hydrogen peroxide solution. Heat again to boiling. The solution should become colorless; if not, repeat the addition of the hydrogen peroxide and the boiling.

6. After decolorization, boil the solution gently for about two minutes. Cool and dilute to 2 ml. mark with distilled water. Mix well by inversion.

7. Transfer 400 lambdas of diluted solution to a 2 ml. test tube.

8. Add 100 lambdas gum-ghatti solution and mix.

9. Add 100 lambdas of the Koch-McMeekin Nessler reagent, mix, and read the optical density on the Beckman DU spectrophotometer against distilled water at 480 mμ.

Calibration

Reagent blank:

1. Transfer 250 lambdas of protein precipitating reagent into a pyrex test tube graduated at 2 ml.

2. Add 25 lambdas of diluted sulfuric acid and dilute to the 2 ml. mark with distilled water.

3. Transfer 400 lambdas of the diluted solution to a 2 ml. test tube.

4. Add 100 lambdas gum-ghatti solution.

5. Add 100 lambdas of the Nessler's reagent and mix well.

The value of the blank in this procedure includes the ammonia present in the reagents.

Since the blank has ordinarily low optical density and is quite constant, it is satisfactory to determine it once for a given lot of reagents and to read future unknowns against distilled water, subtracting the value of the reagent blank from each unknown reading in order to obtain the true reading of the unknown.

Standard:

Use Versatol or any other suitable standard, running it together with each set of unknowns.

This procedure is satisfactory up to 80 mg. NPN/100 ml. serum. If the value is higher than this, the determination should be repeated on a diluted portion of the protein-free supernatant.

Calculation

$$\frac{\text{Value of standard in mg./100 ml.} \times (\text{OD unknown} - \text{OD blank})}{\text{OD standard} - \text{OD blank}}$$
$$= \text{Mg./100 ml. NPN in unknown}$$

Normal Values

Infants and children: 10-30 mg./100 ml. serum
Adults: 29-43 mg./100 ml. whole blood

Discussion

Non-protein nitrogen is present in blood in a number of substances; these include urea (10-17 mg./100 ml.), amino acids (3.4-5.0 mg./100 ml.), uric acid (1.5-2.0 mg./100 ml.), creatinine (0.6-1.2 mg./100 ml.), and lesser amounts in glutathione, ergothioneine, ammonia, indican, and various nucleotides.[2-5] In general, conditions causing elevated blood urea nitrogen also cause retention of other nitrogenous substances and there is a resultant rise in the NPN. NPN and BUN cannot always be used interchangeably, however. In conditions in which there is liver damage (e.g., eclampsia, terminal nephritis), the liver does not make urea and there is a relatively higher elevation of blood non-protein nitrogen than blood urea nitrogen. Parallel serial determinations of NPN and BUN, as advocated by Natelson, will obviously be valuable in assessing deterioration of liver function. Other micro and ultramicro methods are described in the literature.[6, 7]

At birth, concentrations of total non-protein nitrogen are approximately the same in both mother and infant, indicating free diffusion of nitrogen-containing substances across the placenta. In the neonatal period the level is a little higher.[8] In azotemia, values may reach 300 to 400 mg./100 ml; up to 90 per cent of this total may be due to urea. In the absence of liver failure, NPN = 10 + 1.07 × urea N.

REFERENCES

1. KOCH, F. C., AND McMEEKIN, T. L.: *J. Am. Chem. Soc. 46:* 2066, 1924.
2. KING, E. J., AND WOOTTON, I. D. P.: Micro-Analysis in Medical Biochemistry. 3rd Ed., New York, Grune & Stratton, 1956.
3. NATELSON, S.: Microtechniques of Clinical Chemistry for the Routine Laboratory. Springfield, Ill., Charles C Thomas, 1957.
4. GROLLMAN, A.: *Clinical Physiology*—The Functional Pathology of Disease. New York, McGraw-Hill, 1957.
5. BEACH, E. F.: Non-protein nitrogen. *In* Standard Methods of Clinical Chemistry. Vol. 2. New York, Academic Press, 1958.
6. KAPLAN, S. A., AND DEL CARMEN, F. T.: *Pediatrics 17:* 857, 1956.
7. SPIVEK, M. L.: *J. Pediat. 48:* 581, 1956.
8. WOLMAN, I. J.: Laboratory Applications in Clinical Pediatrics. New York, McGraw-Hill, 1957.

16

Inorganic Phosphate

Principle

The proteins in serum are precipitated with trichloroacetic acid and the protein-free filtrate treated with ammonium molybdate. The phosphomolybdic acid formed is reduced by p-semidine hydrochloride to form a "molybdenum blue" complex. The intensity of this blue color is compared with a standard treated in a similar manner.

Apparatus

Pipet, KMP or other ultramicro type, 20 lambdas
Pipet, KMP or other ultramicro type, 25 lambdas
Pipet, KMP or other ultramicro type, 100 lambdas
Pipet, KMP or other ultramicro type, 200 lambdas
Centrifuge, tubes, micro, 1.0 ml.
Test tubes, 7 × 70 mm.

Reagents

1. *Trichloroacetic acid, concentrated:* Dissolve 100 Gm. reagent quality crystalline trichloroacetic acid in distilled water and dilute to 100 ml. This reagent will keep indefinitely if stored in a pyrex glass-stoppered bottle.

2. *Trichloroacetic acid, 10 per cent:* Dilute 10 ml. of concentrated trichloroacetic acid to 100 ml. with distilled water. Store in a pyrex glass-stoppered bottle and prepare fresh each week.

3. *Ammonium molybdate, 0.0083 M.:* Dissolve 2.566 Gm. of ammonium molybdate, $(NH_4)_6Mo_7O_{24} \cdot 4H_2O$, in 250 ml. of water containing 0.25 ml. of concentrated sulfuric acid. This reagent should be stored in a polyethylene bottle.

4. *P-semidine reagent:* Weigh 50 mg. of p-semidine (N-phenyl-p-phenylene-diamine monohydrochloride, EK 2043) and transfer to a dry 100 ml. volu-

metric flask. Wet the solid salt with a few drops of 95 per cent ethanol. Dilute to volume with a 1 per cent solution of sodium bisulfite, $NaHSO_3$. Filter off any insoluble residue. The solution will remain clear for at least 10 days stored at room temperature in a clear glass bottle. After this a slight coloration may appear which does not impair the effectiveness of the reagent, but which will increase the blank absorbence.

5. *Stock phosphorus standard, 1 mg. per ml.:* Weigh about 1 Gm. of reagent quality anhydrous dibasic potassium phosphate (KH_2PO_4), dry overnight in a 110-120 C. oven and cool in a desiccator. Transfer 0.4392 Gm. of this dried compound to a 100 ml. flask and dilute to volume with 5N sulfuric acid. Mix thoroughly.

Procedure

1.   Pipet 200 lambdas of 10 per cent trichloroacetic acid into each of two 1 ml. centrifuge tubes. Label one tube *sample* and the other *blank*.

2.   Add 25 lambdas of serum to the sample tube, and 25 lambdas of distilled water to the blank tube. Mix by running base of tube gently back and forth over a wire test tube rack, or by use of a mixer.

3.   Allow to stand for 5 minutes, centrifuge for 5-10 minutes.

4.   Transfer 100 lambdas of the clear supernatants to similarly labeled 7 × 70 mm. test tubes. Add 20 lambdas of the molybdate reagent to each tube and mix by gently tapping.

5.   Add 200 lambdas of p-semidine reagent to each tube and mix. Allow to stand at room temperature for 10 minutes.

6.   Read the optical density of each tube in a Beckman Spectrophotometer at 700 mμ using distilled water to set the instrument at 100 per cent transmittance.

Calculation

OD sample − OD blank × F = mg. per 100 ml. inorganic phosphorus.
See *Calibration* for F.

Calibration

1. Prepare a dilute standard phosphorus solution by diluting 10 ml. of stock standard to 100 ml. with 10 per cent trichloroacetic acid.

2. Prepare working standards as follows:

Dilute   5 ml. to 25 ml. (with 10 per cent TCA)   =   2 mg. per 100 ml.
10 ml. to 25 ml.   =   4 mg. per 100 ml.

15 ml. to 25 ml.	= 6 mg. per 100 ml.
20 ml. to 25 ml.	= 8 mg. per 100 ml.
Undiluted dilute std.	= 10 mg. per 100 ml.

3. Transfer 25 lambdas of each to 7 × 70 mm. test tubes. Transfer 25 lambdas distilled water to another tube labelled *blank*. Add 200 lambdas 10 per cent trichloroacetic acid to each and mix well. Transfer 100 lambdas of each to a 7 × 70 mm. test tube, and continue with step 4 under *Procedure*.

4. Factor $(F) = \dfrac{\text{equivalent mg. per 100 ml. P}}{\text{OD standard} - \text{OD blank}}$

5. A calibration curve should be plotted to determine the extent of linearity. The mean of the F values is determined and used as a factor for calculating daily determinations. A control specimen should be analyzed with each set of determinations.

Normal Values

Adults: 3-4.5 mg. per 100 ml. serum
Children: 4-6 mg. per 100 ml. serum
    (*See* Discussion)

Discussion

This is a modification of the method of Dryer, Tammes, and Routh.[1] Most methods for the analysis of serum inorganic phosphorus depend on the reduction of phosphomolybdic acid, but differ in their choice of reducing agents. The most commonly used reagent is 1-amino-2-naphthol-4-sulfonic acid,[2] but this is not satisfactory for ultramicro use because of low absorbances. Stannous chloride[3] is not recommended because the absorbances are not constant with respect to time and the reagent is not stable. The use of Elon[4] as the reducing agent requires 45 minutes or more to develop maximum color. The present method using p-semidine gives adequate absorbances for ultramicro analysis and the reagent is relatively stable. The maximum color is developed in 5-10 minutes and remains unchanged for at least 1.5 hours.

Dryer, Tammes and Routh found maximum absorbances of this reaction at 350 and 770 mμ. The 700 mμ wavelength recommended here is more satisfactory with most spectrophotometers, but greater sensitivity will be obtained at the other wavelengths, particularly the one in the ultraviolet region.

Contamination is a problem often encountered in ultramicro serum phosphorus methods. Detergents and many reagents will leave sufficient residual phosphate on the surface of the glassware to cause erroneous results. Commercial heparin preparations have been reported to be heavily contaminated with phosphorus.[5] It is best to maintain a separate set of glassware for use only with this method. The use of a regular control specimen is recommended. Either previously analyzed pooled serum or Lab-Trol may be used.

Normal values for serum inorganic phosphorus were studied by Greenburg, Winters and Graham.[6] Regression curves of serum phosphorus on age were fitted to a large number of normal observations. They found that sex as well as age affected the normal value. Curves for both male and female at age one year indicated a phosphorus level of about 5 mg. per 100 ml., the curve for females being somewhat higher than males. Their curve for males fell steadily and progressively for the first three decades, after which it gradually flattened out, and after age 70 showed a slight upturn. Their curve for females showed a steeper fall than the male curve during the earlier decades, reaching a definite minimum at about age 45. After this there was a slight progressive upturn. Young,[7] using the Fiske and SubbaRow method, reported values in adult blood donors of 2.4-4.7 Gm. per 100 ml., 89 per cent of these falling between 3.2 and 4.3 mg. per 100 ml.

Serum inorganic phosphorus is higher in summer than in winter due to the increased concentration of solar ultraviolet rays. The phosphorus level will vary with carbohydrate utilization due to the part played by phosphorylation. Serum phosphorus falls gradually after ingestion of carbohydrate and returns to normal within 4-5 hours. This is independent of the blood sugar level. Annino reported a small but significant drop in phosphorus levels 45 minutes after eating breakfast.[8] In diabetes this phosphorus response is either diminished or does not occur. There will be a slight decrease in the inorganic phosphorus level after ingestion of calcium.

Kyle reports that variations in serum phosphorus levels occur during the day, with lowest levels during the early morning hours.[9]

Infants under one year will have phosphorus levels influenced by such other variables as dietary phosphorus load, and renal or parathyroid immaturity.[10-14]

Serum inorganic phosphorus rises in severe nephritis (so-called phosphate retention). Values above 8 mg. per 100 ml. are important for prognosis of the patient's condition. There is a slight elevation (5-7 mg. per 100 ml.) during bone healing and in hypoparathyroidism (proportional to the decrease in calcium). Hyperphosphatemia also occurs in multiple myeloma, tuberculosis, malignant disease, renal rickets, hypervitaminosis D, uremia and acute high intestinal obstruction.

Hypophosphatemia occurs in rickets and after insulin or epinephrine injection; in osteomalacia, ideopathic steatorrhea, hyperparathyroidism, sprue, lobar pneumonia, myxedema, and during ether, chloroform or ethylene anesthesia.

REFERENCES

1. DRYER, R. L., TAMMES, A. R., AND ROUTH, J. I.: *J. Biol. Chem. 225:* 177, 1957.
2. FISKE, C. H., AND SUBBAROW, Y.: *J. Biol. Chem. 66:* 375, 1925.
3. KUTTNER, T., AND COHEN, H. R.: *J. Biol. Chem. 75:* 517, 1927.
4. GOMORI, G.: *J. Lab. & Clin. Med. 27:* 955, 1941-42.
5. MCGEOWN, M. G., MARTIN, E., AND NEILL, D. W.: *J. Clin. Path. 8:* 247, 1955.
6. GREENBURG, B. G., WINTERS, R. W., AND GRAHAM, J. G.: *J. Clin. Endocrinol. 20:* 364, 1960.
7. YOUNG, N. F.: *In* Standard Methods of Clinical Chemistry, Vol. I, Reiner, M., ed., New York, Academic Press, 1953.
8. ANNINO, J. S., AND RELMAN, A. S.: *Am. J. Clin. Path. 31:* 155, 1959.
9. KYLE, L. H., SCHAAF, M., AND CANARY, J. J.: *Am. J. Med. 24:* 240, 1958.
10. TODD, W. R., CHUINARD, E. G., AND WOOD, M. T.: *Am. J. Dis. Child. 57:* 1278, 1939.
11. BARNES, D. J., AND MUNKS, B.: *Proc. Soc. Exper. Biol. & Med. 44:* 327, 1940.
12. GITTELMAN, I. F., AND PINCUS, J. B.: *Pediatrics 8:* 778, 1954.
13. GRAHAM, G. C., BARNESS, L. A., AND GYÖRGY, R.: *J. Pediat. 42:* 401, 1953.
14. BRUCK, E., AND WEINTRAUB, D. H.: *A.M.A. Am. J. Dis. Child. 90:* 653, 1955.

17

Acid and Alkaline Phosphatase

Principle

Disodium monophenyl phosphate is used as a substrate to determine the activity of either acid or alkaline phosphatase.[1] Serum is incubated at 37 C. with the substrate in a solution buffered to pH 10.0 or pH 4.9—the optimum conditions for either enzyme using the buffers in this procedure. After hydrolysis, which liberates phenol, the protein is precipitated with the Folin-Ciocalteu reagent.[2] Sodium carbonate is then added to develop a blue color. This color is a complex formed when the phosphotungstate and phosphomolybdate are allowed to react with a reducing agent, such as the phenol which was formed by the enzyme. The King-Armstrong unit is defined as the activity per 100 ml. of serum which will liberate 1 mg. of phenol from the buffered disodium monophenyl phosphate under the conditions of the test. These are converted to approximate Bodansky units by dividing the King-Amstrong units by two.

Apparatus

Pipet, KMP or other ultramicro type, 25 lambdas
Pipet, KMP or other ultramicro type, 250 lambdas
Pipet, KMP or other ultramicro type, 500 lambdas
Test tubes, 7 x 70 mm.
Centrifuge tubes, Micro, 1 ml.
Water bath, 37 C.

Reagents

1. *Disodium phenyl phosphate, 0.01M:*[3] Weigh 2.18 Gm. of reagent quality disodium monophenyl phosphate and transfer to a one-liter volumetric flask. Dissolve in distilled water and dilute to mark. Sterilize by transferring the solution to a beaker and bringing it quickly to the boiling point. Cool im-

mediately, transfer to a glass-stoppered pyrex bottle, add a few drops of chloroform, and store in the refrigerator.

2. *Alkaline buffer, pH 10.0:*[3] Transfer 6.36 Gm. of anhydrous sodium carbonate (Na_2CO_3) and 3.36 Gm. of sodium bicarbonate ($NaHCO_3$) to a one-liter volumetric flask. Add approximately 500 ml. of distilled water, mix to dissolve, dilute to mark with distilled water and mix. Store in a glass-stoppered bottle in the refrigerator. The pH of the solution should be checked, preferably on a pH meter.

3. *Acid buffer, pH 49:*[3] Dissolve 21.0 Gm. of reagent quality crystalline citric acid monohydrate ([$HOCCOOH(CH_3COOH)_2 \cdot H_2O$]) in 200 ml. distilled water in a 500 ml. volumetric flask. Add 188 ml. of 1N sodium hydroxide (standardized), and dilute to volume. The pH of this solution should be checked on a pH meter, and adjusted if necessary with either 0.1N sodium hydroxide or 0.1N hydrochloric acid. Transfer to a glass-stoppered bottle, add a few drops of chloroform, and store in the refrigerator.

4. *Buffered alkaline substrate:* Mix 50 ml. of substrate (1) with 50 ml. of alkaline buffer (2). Store in refrigerator.

5. *Buffered acid substrate:* Mix 25 ml. of substrate (1) with 25 ml. of acid buffer (3). Store in refrigerator.

6. *Phenol reagent, Folin-Ciocalteu:* Transfer into a two-liter glass-jointed Florence flask 100 Gm. sodium tungstate ($Na_2WO_4 \cdot 2H_2O$), 25 Gm. sodium molybdate ($Na_2MoO_4 \cdot 2H_2O$) and 700 ml. distilled water. Shake to dissolve and add 50 ml. of 85 per cent phosphoric acid and 100 ml. of concentrated hydrochloric acid, mixing thoroughly. Connect the ground glass joint to a reflux condenser, add a few glass beads and boil gently for 10 hours. After removing condenser, add 150 Gm. lithium sulfate (Li_2SO_4) and 50 ml. of bromine water or 50 ml. distilled water plus a few drops of liquid bromine. Boil the mixture without a condenser for at least 15 minutes to remove the excess bromine. There should be no green color, but a clear golden yellow. If the reagent is green, add more bromine water and repeat the process. Cool to room temperature, dilute to one liter with distilled water and filter. This reagent will keep for several months in a well-stoppered brown bottle. Before use, dilute 1 part phenol reagent with 2 parts distilled water. A commercially prepared reagent may be preferred.

7. *Phenol stock standard, 1 mg. per ml.:* This reagent requires a rather lengthy method of standardization. It is usually best to obtain it from a commercial source such as the Hartman-Leddon Co. However, it may be prepared as follows:

a. Weigh approximately 1.2 Gm. reagent quality crystalline phenol and transfer to a one-liter volumetric flask. Dissolve in about 800 ml. of 0.1N hydrochloric acid, prepared by diluting 8.5 ml. concentrated HCl to one liter with distilled water. Dilute to mark with 0.1N hydrochloric acid. Keeps indefinitely after standarization at refrigerator temperature.

b. *Standardization:* Transfer 25 ml. of this solution to a 250 ml. glass-stoppered Erlenmeyer flask. Add 50 ml. of 0.1N sodium hydroxide and heat to 65 C. While mixing, add 25 ml. of 0.1N iodine solution, stopper and allow to stand at room temperature for 30-40 minutes. Next add 5 ml. concentrated hydrochloric acid and titrate the excess of iodine with 0.1N sodium thiosulfate solution. When the iodine color has faded to a pale yellow, add 1 ml. of 1 per cent soluble starch and titrate until the blue starch-iodine color disappears. Each ml. of 0.1N iodine solution used (25 ml. minus the ml. of thiosulfate used) as equivalent to 1.567 mg. phenol.

1.567 × (ml. 0.1N I_2 − ml. 0.1N $Na_2S_2O_3$ used) = mg. phenol per 25 ml.

Adjust this concentration to 1 mg. per ml. by dilution with 0.1N hydrochloric acid.

c. Sodium thiosulfate 0.1N is prepared by transferring 25 Gm. of reagent quality sodium thiosulfate ($Na_2S_2O_3 \cdot 5H_2O$) to a liter flask and dissolving in about 700 ml. of freshly boiled and cooled distilled water. Dilute to mark and allow to stand two weeks. Standardize this solution with 0.1N solution of acid potassium iodate $KH(IO_3)_2$ ([3.2496 Gm. reagent quality $KH(IO_3)_2$ diluted to one liter with distilled water]). Place 1 Gm. of reagent quality potassium iodide in a 500 ml. Erlenmeyer flask and dissolve in as little water as possible. Add 5 ml. of 20 per cent HCl and 25 ml. of the 0.1N KH $(IO_3)_2$, dilute to 200 ml. with distilled water and rapidly titrate the liberated iodine with the sodium thiosulfate solution. When the solution becomes pale yellow, add 2 ml. of 1 per cent soluble starch solution and titrate until the blue color disappears. Dilute the thiosulfate as follows:

$$\frac{25}{\text{ml. thiosulfate used}} = \frac{X}{\text{volume of remaining thiosulfate}}$$

X = Final volume of thiosulfate

d. *Iodine solution, 0.1N:* Transfer 25 Gm. reagent quality potassium iodide to a one-liter volumetric flask and dissolve in about 250 ml. of distilled water. Add 12.7 Gm. powdered resublimed iodine and dissolve. Store in a glass-stoppered brown bottle. To standardize this solution, transfer 25 ml. of the iodine solution to a 250 ml. Erlenmeyer flask and add 100 ml. of distilled water. Titrate with 0.1N sodium thiosulfate until the solution becomes pale yellow, then add 1 ml. of a 1 per cent solution of soluble starch and titrate drop by drop until the blue color disappears. Calculate the normality of the iodine solution and adjust to 0.1N.

8. *Phenol working standard, 0.02 mg. per ml.:* Dilute 2.0 ml. phenol stock standard to 100 ml. with distilled water. This solution is stable at least three months in the refrigerator.

Procedure

Alkaline Phosphatase:
1. Place 25 lambdas of serum into a 1 ml. centrifuge tube (A).
2. Add 500 lambdas buffered substrate (either acid or alkaline as required) and mix by gentle tapping or by running the base of the test tube gently back and forth over a wire test tube rack.
3. Incubate at 37 C. for exactly 15 minutes. During the final 5 minutes, place 500 lambdas buffered substrate into another 1 ml. centrifuge tube for a reagent blank (B).
4. After incubation *immediately* add 500 lambdas of dilute phenol reagent to all tubes.
5. Add 25 lambdas of serum to reagent tube B. Mix all tubes and centrifuge for 5 minutes.
6. Transfer 500 lambdas of the clear supernatant from each tube to a 7 × 70 mm. test tube similarly labeled.
7. Add 250 lambdas of 20 per cent sodium carbonate to each tube. Note time of addition, mix and allow each tube to stand *exactly* 20 minutes.
8. Transfer to micro cuvets just before the end of the 20 minutes. At the end of the time period, read the optical density in a Beckman DU spectrophotometer at 660 mμ, setting the instrument at 100 per cent transmittance with distilled water.

Acid Phosphatase:

Use buffered acid substrate and incubate for 1 hour.

Calculation

OD "A" − OD "B" × F = phosphatase in King'Armstrong units per 100 ml. of serum.

Calibration

1. Dilute 1.0, 2.0, 3.0 and 10.0 ml. of phenol working standard to 10.0 ml. with distilled water and mix. In this method, these diluted standards are equivalent to serum phosphatase values of 4.1, 8.2, 12.3, and 41.0 units per 100 ml. based on a 1:21 dilution of the original serum.
2. Pipet 525 lambdas of each standard into appropriately labeled 7 × 70 mm. test tubes. Pipet 525 lambdas distilled water into a fifth tube for a reagent blank.

3. Add 500 lambdas of dilute phenol reagent to each tube.

4. Continue with step 6 given under *Procedure*.

5. Plot the optical density against King-Armstrong unit equivalents for each standard. This chart may be used for daily determinations by obtaining values for both incubated (A) and unincubated samples (B) and subtracting B from A. If the graph shows good conformance to Beer's Law, a factor (F) for calculating daily analyses may be determined as follows:

$$F = \frac{\text{equivalent KA units/100 ml. serum.}}{\text{OD "A"} - \text{OD "B"}}$$

Normal Values

Alkaline phosphatase:	*Adults* to 13 King-Armstrong Units
	Children to 20 King-Armstrong Units
Acid phosphatase:	to 5 King-Armstrong Units

Discussion

Serum specimens used for the analysis of acid phosphatase should show no traces of hemolysis since erythrocytes contain large amounts of the enzyme. The serum should be analyzed the same day the blood is drawn. The phosphatase activity in stored blood gradually diminishes. The activity of serum will remain rather constant up to seven days if kept frozen but will decline rapidly at room temperature. Blood should be withdrawn during the post-absorptive state.

Timing is important during incubation and color development. If a series of samples is to be analyzed consecutively, the sodium carbonate should be added at spaced intervals to permit reading each sample after exactly 20 minutes. If the supernatant is not clear after centrifugation, the tyrosine in the protein will cause falsely elevated values of phosphatase. Use only clear supernatant solution.

Since an elevated acid phosphatase activity is fairly specific for metastasizing carcinoma of the prostate, it is recommended that elevated results be carefully checked by using a fresh specimen of blood. Manipulation of the prostate gland, such as in a physical examination, may cause elevated acid phosphatase levels; it is best to repeat the test after 24 hours whenever an elevated level is found.[4] Slight elevations occasionally occur in prostatitis, benign hypertrophy of the prostate, or carcinoma of the prostate without metastases.

Elevated values for serum alkaline phosphatase are found in pathologic bone metabolism, hepatic and biliary tract disorders, rickets, hyperparathyroidism, multiple myeloma, and many other disorders. It may be decreased in hypothyroidism, celiac disease, and severe chronic nephritis.

Since alkaline phosphatase is involved in active bone formation, higher normal values are found in children. These values are low at birth, rise rapidly to a maximum during the first month of life and remain stable through the second year. They fall to adult normal values during late childhood.

REFERENCES

1. KING, E. J., AND ARMSTRONG, A. R.: *Canad. M. As. J. 31:* 376, 1934.
2. FOLIN, O., AND CIOCALTEU, V.: *J. Biol. Chem. 73:* 627, 1927.
3. CARR, J. J.: Standard Methods of Clinical Chemistry, Vol. I, Reiner, M., ed., New York, Academic Press, Inc., 1953, p. 75.
4. MACDONALD R. P.: *Harper Hosp. Bull. 16:* 77, 1958.

18

Proteins: Total Serum, Serum Albumin and Globulin, and Cerebrospinal Fluid

TOTAL SERUM PROTEIN

Principle

A modified biuret reagent is used to produce a blue color in a solution of serum.[1] The color is then compared with a standard protein solution which has been treated in a similar manner.

Apparatus

Pipet, KMP or other ultramicro type, 25 lambdas
Pipet, volumetric 2 ml.
Test tubes, 13 × 100 mm.

Reagents

1. *Sodium hydroxide, saturated solution:* Carefully dissolve 110 Gm. reagent quality sodium hydroxide pellets in 100 ml. distilled water with constant stirring. Cool and allow to stand one week until sediment settles out. Decant and use clear supernatant solution.

2. *Sodium hydroxide, 10 per cent:* Dilute 42 ml. of the sodium hydroxide solution (1) to 300 ml. with distilled water and mix.

3. *Biuret reagent (Gornall):*[2] Dissolve 1.5 Gm. reagent copper sulfate ($CuSO_4 \cdot 5H_2O$) and 6.0 Gm. sodium-potassium tartrate ($NaKC_4H_4O_6 \cdot 4H_2O$) into 500 ml. distilled water in a one-liter volumetric flask. Add with constant stirring 300 ml. of 10 per cent carbonate-free sodium hydroxide, dilute to mark and mix.

Procedure

1. **Pipet 25 lambdas of serum into a 13 × 100 mm. test tube labeled**

A. For a reagent blank, pipet 25 lambdas of distilled water into another test tube labeled B. A third tube, labeled S, should contain 25 lambdas of a commercially prepared protein standard (e.g., Lab-Trol, Hyland Control Serum, Versatol).

2.   Add 2.0 ml. of biuret reagent to each test tube. Mix by gentle tapping.

3.   Allow to stand at room temperature for 30 minutes.

4.   Measure optical density of the sample, standard, and the reagent blank in a Beckman spectrophotometer at 540 mμ wavelength. Distilled water is used to set the instrument at 100 per cent transmittance.

Calculation

$$\frac{OD_A - OD_B}{OD_S - OD_B} \times \text{Gm./100 ml. protein} = \text{Gm./100 ml. total}$$
$$\text{in standard} \qquad \text{protein}$$

Calibration

This procedure produces a calibration curve which is linear throughout the physiologic range. No calibration curve is required, but the commercial standard being used should be checked against at least one other commercial standard. Commercial standards are usually reliable, but occasionally may be in error.[3] Errors may also occur in reconstitution, or the solution may have been stored for too long a period.

A factor may be calculated as follows:

$$F = \frac{\text{Gm./100 ml. protein}}{OD_S - OD_B}$$

Then $F \times (OD_A - OD_B) = \text{Gm./100 ml. protein in sample}$

Normal Values

> *Total protein:*
> Adult: 6.0—8.0 Gm. per 100 ml.
> Newborn: 5.6—6.6 Gm. per 100 ml.
> Premature: 5.0—6.0 Gm. per 100 ml.

Discussion

Blood for this analysis must be withdrawn during the postabsorptive state. The serum should be separated from the cells as soon as possible and there should be no visible hemolysis. This procedure will produce results comparable to the macro methods employing the biuret reaction. Samples of 10 lambdas of serum may be used if quantities of all reagents are decreased by appropriate amounts. If a commercially prepared protein standard is not available, pooled serum can be used for the calibration. Protein content may be determined by a micro-Kjeldahl procedure.[4]

Serum protein ions contribute to the anion portion of the electrolyte balance. Because at pH 7.4 they are in solution on the alkaline side of their isoelectric points, they exist to a certain extent as alkaline salts. Among their chief functions are the maintenance of normal blood volume and normal tissue water content. Depletion of plasma proteins leads to edema, thereby influencing the entire electrolyte concentration. Palpable edema usually develops when the concentration of serum protein falls below 5 Gm. per 100 ml.

A decrease in plasma protein of 1 Gm. per cent results in a significant change in plasma volume. Blood plasma and interstitial fluid differ primarily in their concentration of nondiffusible protein. The total electrolyte equivalents of plasma is greater than that of interstitial fluid by the base equivalents of plasma protein. Fluid moves from the arteries into the interstitial spaces by heart action. The return flow is provided by the unopposed osmotic differential due to the plasma proteins. This pressure gradient exists because the same quantity of base ion will exert more osmotic pressure when combined with a monovalent ion (e.g. Cl or HCO_3) than it will when combined with a polyvalent protein ion.

The concentration of plasma protein expressed in Gm. per 100 ml. may be converted to milliequivalents by use of the following equation:[5]

$$mEq./L. = 0.104 \ (Gm. \ protein/L.) \ (pH—5.08)$$

Total proteins show a gradual decline from about 6 Gm./100 ml. the first week of life to approximately 4.5 Gm./100 ml. at 30 days.[6] The figures of Mayer, Kelley, et al. are slightly lower.[7] They found the average serum protein levels of white and Negro infants under 10 days of age to be 5.69—5.87 Gm./100 ml., while figures for white and Negro premature infants were 5.60 Gm. and 5.25 Gm./100 ml. respectively. Higher protein levels for term infants as compared with premature infants have been reported by other authors as well.[8-11] The plasma protein level gradually rises during early childhood and reaches adult levels at about five years of age.

The *percentage* of albumin in plasma decreases from infancy and is lowest in the 5-11 year-old group, but figures for the *absolute* concentration of albumin in Gm./100 ml. show no significant decrease in albumin during this period.[12] Albumin is decreased in anemia, carcinoma, edema, glomerulonephritis, hemorrhage, infections, leukemia, liver disease, malnutrition, and nephrosis. Globulin is increased in multiple myeloma and is increased to the extent albumin is decreased in several other disorders. Discussion of relative changes in the globulin fraction will be found in the chapter on *Electrochromatography.*

SERUM ALBUMIN AND GLOBULIN

Principle

The serum globulins are salted out with a solution of 23 per cent sodium sulfate. Total protein and albumin are determined individually by the biuret reaction, and globulin calculated as the total protein minus albumin.

Apparatus

Pipet, KMP or other ultramicro type, 25 lambdas
Pipet, KMP or other ultramicro type, 100 lambdas
Pipet, KMP or other ultramicro type, 250 or 500 lambdas
Centrifuge tube, 1 ml. micro.
Test tube, 7 × 70 mm.

Reagents

1. *Sodium sulfate, 23 per cent:* Dissolve 23.0 Gm. reagent quality anhydrous sodium sulfate with distilled water in a 100 ml. volumetric flask and dilute to mark. This may crystallize out if the room temperature becomes too cold. If this occurs, store the reagent at 37 C. until the solution clears.

2. *Span-ether:[13]* Add 1 ml. Span 20 (Atlas Powder Co., Wilmington, Del.) to 99 ml. of ether and mix well. Filter through Whatman No. 1 filter paper. Make up to 100 ml. volume with ether. Store in glass-stoppered bottle.

3. *Biuret reagent: (See under Total Protein.)*

Procedure

1. Pipet 25 lambdas of serum into a 1 ml. centrifuge tube. Add 500 lambdas (using 250 lambda pipet twice) of 23 per cent sodium sulfate and mix by gentle tapping.

2. Add about 0.5 ml. of span-ether, place clean finger over the mouth of the tube and shake for about 30 seconds (*caution when using ether*). Centrifuge for 2 or 3 minutes.

3. Remove carefully 100 lambdas of the albumin layer by folding the rubber aspirator tubing just above the pipet tip, slanting the centrifuge tube so that the globulin layer is free of the sides of the tube, and then cautiously place the pipet tip under the globulin layer. *No span-ether should enter the pipet.* Withdraw liquid to the 100 lambda mark. Remove the pipet from the solution and wipe off adhering globulin particles while holding the pipet nearly horizontal.

4.   Transfer to a 7 × 70 mm. test tube marked **A**. Place 100 lambdas of 23 per cent sodium sulfate into another test tube marked **B** for the reagent blank.

5.   Pipet 200 lambdas of biuret reagent into each tube, mix by gentle tapping and allow to stand at room temperature *for 30 minutes*.

6.   Measure optical density of the sample and reagent blank in a Beckman spectrophotometer at 540 mμ. Distilled water is used to set the instrument at 100 per cent transmittance.

Calculation

$$(OD_A—OD_B) \times F = Gm. \text{ per 100 ml. albumin.}$$

The Gm. per 100 ml. globulin is calculated by subtracting Gm. per 100 ml. albumin from Gm. per 100 ml. total protein.

The albumin to globulin ratio (A/G) is obtained by dividing Gm. per 100 ml. albumin by Gm. per 100 ml. globulin.

Calibration

The calibration factor for albumin is derived from the factor used to calculate total protein. The final serum dilution for the albumin method is 1:63, for the total protein method it is 1:81; thus the factor used to calculate albumin is:

$$\text{Albumin factor} = \text{total protein factor} \times \frac{63}{81}$$

Normal Values

Adults:
Albumin: 3.5—5.6 Gm./100 ml.
Globulin: 1.3—3.2 Gm./100 ml.
A/G Ratio: 1.5—2.5/1

Normal Children:[12]

Age	Albumin	A/G Ratio
6-46 weeks	3.92	1.56/1
1-4 years	4.37	1.56/1
5-11 years	4.23	1.32/1
13-17 years	4.40	1.54/1

Discussion

All precautions for the total protein method apply to albumin. Too vigorous shaking of the serum-salt mixture with span-ether should be avoided to prevent the possibility of denaturing the albumin.[14] However, too little shaking will result in incomplete separation of the globulin and lead to falsely high albumin values.

CEREBROSPINAL FLUID PROTEIN

Principle

Protein in cerebrospinal fluid is determined using the Folin phenol reagent and alkaline copper reagent.[15] There is an initial biuret type of reaction between the protein and copper in alkali, then a reduction of the phosphotungstic-phosphomolybdic acids of the reagent by both the copper-protein complex and by the tyrosine and tryptophane of the protein.

Apparatus

Pipet, KMP or other ultramicro type, 25 lambdas
Pipet, KMP or other ultramicro type, 50 lambdas
Pipet, serologic, 5.0 ml.
Test tube, 15 × 85 mm.

Reagents

1. *Alkaline carbonate:* Dissolve 20 Gm. sodium carbonate, Na_2CO_3 and 0.5 Gm. sodium *or* potassium tartrate, $Na_2C_4H_4O_6 \cdot 2H_2O$ or $K_2C_4H_4O_6 \cdot \frac{1}{2}H_2O$, in a liter of 0.1 N NaOH.

2. *Copper sulfate, 0.1 per cent:* Transfer 1 Gm. of copper sulfate, $CuSO_4 \cdot 5H_2O$, to a one-liter flask, dissolve in distilled water and dilute to mark.

3. *Working alkaline copper reagent:* Mix 9 ml. of (1) with 5 ml. of (2). Prepare daily.

4. *Dilute Folin-Ciocalteu reagent:* Titrate 1 ml. of Folin and Ciocalteu reagent (*see under Phosphatase*) plus 50 ml. of distilled water to a phenolphthalein end-point using 0.1 N NaOH. On the basis of this titration dilute the reagent so that 1 ml. is equivalent to 9.0 ml. of 0.1 N NaOH. A dilution to about one-half strength will be required.

    Example: Titration = 19.8 ml.

        To make 500 ml.: Divide titration by 2 (9.9) because the stock phenol reagent will be twice as concentrated as the working reagent.

$$\frac{500}{9.9} \times \frac{x}{9.0} = 9.9 \times 4500 = 445$$

Therefore, dilute 445 ml. of the reagent to 500 ml. with distilled water.

5. *Working phenol reagent:*   Add 1 part of (4) to 1 part of distilled water.

6. *Protein standard:*   Determine the protein content of a sample of normal human serum by a Kjeldahl method, or use a commercial protein standard. Dilute this serum with 0.85 per cent NaCl to a level of 40 mg. per cent protein. This may be preserved with benzoic acid, *never thymol.*

Procedure

1.   Transfer 2.5 ml. of alkaline copper reagent to each of three 15 x 85 mm. test tubes. Label these tubes blank, unknown, and standard.

2.   Add 50 lambdas of cerebrospinal fluid to the "unknown" tube, 50 lambdas of protein standard to the "standard" tube, and 50 lambdas of distilled water to the "blank" tube.

3.   Mix and allow to stand at room temperature for 15 minutes.

4.   Add RAPIDLY *(Important!),* with constant mixing, 25 lambdas of working phenol reagent to each tube. Blowing air through the pipet and stirring with the tip of the pipet will aid in rapid mixing.

5.   After 30 minutes, transfer to ultramicro cuvets and read the optical density in a spectrophotometer at 660 mμ wavelength. Set the instrument at 100 per cent transmittance using the reagent blank.

6.   The test is best performed in duplicate.

7.   For very high cerebrospinal fluid protein levels, repeat the test using diluted cerebrospinal fluid. However, reasonably good results will be obtained in an emergency by diluting the final colored solution with distilled water, and using the appropriate dilution factor in the calculation. The final color is stable about three hours.

Calculation

$$\left[\frac{OD \ unk.}{OD \ std.} \times 40 \right] - 6^* = \text{mg. per 100 ml. protein in CSF}$$

Normal Value

Adults: 15-45 mg. per 100 ml. protein.
Children: 15-55 mg. per 100 ml. protein.

---

*6 mg. per cent is subtracted from the result to correct for the average color value of the non-protein substances taking part in the reaction.

CALIBRATION CURVE FOR SPINAL FLUID PROTEINS
(Beckman DU 660 mμ[15]) (Daughady, Lowry et al.)

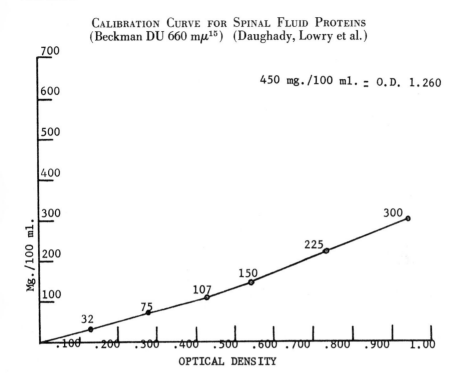

450 mg./100 ml. $\div$ O.D. 1.260

Discussion

The cerebrospinal fluid should first be centrifuged to remove any cells or pellicle, and only clear fluid used for protein analysis.

At pH 10, which is the optimal pH for color development, the Folin-Ciocalteu reagent remains active for only a few seconds. It is for this reason that special emphasis is given to the rapidity with which the reagent is added. The 15 x 85 mm. tubes are also recommended for this reason. The precision of the method is excellent when attention is given to this detail.

This combination of a buiret and "tyrosine equivalences" method is highly sensitive. The color from non-protein substances is quite constant, and should not vary more than 2 mg. per cent from a mean value of 6 mg. per cent.[15] Sethna and Tsao [16] report that a "tyrosine equivalence" method will give good results regardless of the A/G ratio, even though the color from a given amount of globulin is slightly more intense than that which would be obtained from the same amount of albumin. They state this error will not change the results appreciably.

Various drugs have been reported to cause erroneously high values using this method.[17] These drugs include salicylates, chlorpromazine, chloramphenicol, tyrosine, many sulfa drugs, penicillin, streptomycin, and terramycin. In cases of suspected drug interference a protein-free filtrate should be prepared and its absorbence subtracted from the absorbence obtained from the diluted protein.

REFERENCES

1. KINGSLEY, G. R.: *J. Biol. Chem. 131:* 197, 1939.
2. GORNALL, A. G., BARDAWILL, C. J., AND DAVID, M. M.: *J. Biol. Chem. 177:* 751, 1949.
3. REMP, D. G.: Personal communication.
4. ARCHIBALD, R. M.: *In* Standard Methods of Clinical Chemistry, Vol. II, Seligson, D., ed., New York, Academic Press, Inc., 1958, p. 91.
5. VAN SLYKE, D. D., HASTINGS, A. B., HILLER, A., AND SENDROY, J.: *Biol. Chem. 79:* 769, 1928.
6. NORTON, P. M., KUNZ H., AND PRATT, E. L.: *Pediatrics 10:* 527, 1952.
7. MOYER, E. Z., KELLY, H. J., MACY I. G., MACK H. C., DI LORETO, P. C., AND PRATT, J. P.: Nutritional Status of Mothers and Their Infants. Detroit, The Children's Fund of Michigan, 1954.
8. SMITH, C. A.: The Physiology of the Newborn Infant, 2nd ed., Springfield, Ill., Charles C Thomas, 1951.
9. MCMURRAY, L. G., ROE, J. H., AND SWEET, L. K.: *Am. J. Dis. Child. 75:* 265, 1948.
10. STERNBERG, S. D., AND GREENBLATT, I. J.: *Allergy Ann. 9:* 204, 1951.
11. DARROW, D. C., AND CARY, M. K.: *J. Pediat. 3:* 573, 1933.
12. KNAPP, E. L., AND ROUTH, J. I.: *Pediatrics 4:* 508, 1949.
13. WOLFSON, W. Q., COHN, C., CALVARY, E., AND ICHIBA F.: *Am. J. Clin. Path. 18:* 723, 1948.
14. SAIFER, A., AND ZYMARIS M. C.: *Clin. Chem. 1:* 180, 1955.
15. DAUGHADAY, W. H., LOWRY, O. H., ROSEBROUGH, N. J., AND FIELDS, W. S.: *J. Lab. & Clin. Med. 39:* 662, 1952.
16. SETHNA, S., AND TSAO, M. U.: *Clin. Chem. 3:* 249, 1957.
17. ZONDAG, H. A., AND VAN BOETZELAER, G. L.: *Clin. Chem. Acta 8:* 121, 1960.

19

Electrochromatography

Principle

Few fields attract as much interest today as chromatography and electrochromatography. New articles are being published on these subjects at the rate of a thousand a year. But in spite of the plethora of accumulated data on the dynamics of differential migration, how they are affected by driving and opposing forces remains poorly understood. It is perhaps best to preface this discussion then with some fundamental definitions, and those of Strain and Sato[1] seem particularly appropriate.

1. Chromatographic analysis is a differential migration technic in which the flow of solvent or gas causes the components of mixtures to migrate differentially from a narrow initial zone in a porous sorptive medium.

2. Electrochromatographic analysis is a differential migration technic in which direct current electrical potential causes the components of mixtures to migrate differentially from a narrow initial zone in a stabilized background electrolytic solution.

3. Continuous electrochromatographic analysis is a differential migration technic in which the flow of background electrolytic solution through a wide porous medium and a transverse direct current potential causes the components of mixtures to migrate differentially from a narrow continuous stream of solution flowing continuously with the background electrolytic solution.

Paper electrophoresis as applied to the clinical laboratory remains largely empirical in nature. The reason for this is the large number of variables with which one must contend. Ionized substances may become converted into unionized complexes or into ionized complexes with either the same or opposite electrical charge. Slight changes in pH, solvent electric potential, humidity, temperature, sorbent, timing and the technologist's frame of mind all affect the separability. The staining methods may still further alter the interpretation.

Paper electrophoresis apparatus can be classified as follows:[2]

Paper suspended in a vapor space: To avoid a disturbing effect from supports, many designs use a paper strip suspended between widely-spaced supports. The horizontally-hanging strip will be curved with the center lower than the ends, and this may cause the pooling of buffer at the center of the strips. Only a limited amount of tension can be applied at the ends of the strips because of the weakness of wet paper. In other designs the paper is supported in the center, forming an inverted V. This decreases the effect of the buffer pooling at the center but introduces gravitational effects. The sample is applied at the tip and migration takes place down one side of the inverted V.

Paper supported in a vapor space: The paper is maintained in an accurate horizontal position by plastic spikes or bristles. The paper rests on the spike tips with only a very small area coming into contact with it.

Apparatus without a vapor space: The disturbing factor of water evaporation from paper surfaces, especially when high voltage is used, is eliminated in this method. In one design the paper is placed in a non-conducting liquid. (Chlorobenzene has been used.) The suspending liquid may affect the electrophoresis process and it is technically complicated to maintain a proper liquid bath. Another type has two glass or plastic pressure plates with or without liquid cooling systems, and the paper is pressed uniformly between them. Unfortunately, water temperatures in hospitals are often subject to considerable variability and may not provide as constant a temperature as mechanical or gas refrigeration.

A starch-supporting medium for zone electrophoresis has also proven useful in the separation of protein mixtures. Since its introduction by Kunkel and Slater[3] for the study of lipoproteins in serum, it has been used in the analysis of bacterial enzymes,[4] virus inhibitors,[5] serum proteins,[6] human hemoglobins,[7-9] and separation of antibodies.[10]

Apparatus

Paper electrophoresis apparatus may be constructed according to the principles given above[11-15] or purchased in any of several designs. We have used the LKB and the Spinco electrophoresis apparatus described in the chapter on *Special Equipment.* The LKB instrument utilizes the horizontal filter paper strips supported on spikes and is used in a large refrigerator for temperature control; the Spinco is of the inverted V design.

Densitometers are also discussed in the chapter on *Special Equipment* and are available in either the automatic or semiautomatic form. The Photovolt densitometer, Model 425, is a semi-automatic instrument which is satisfactory for handling a moderate work load. (Photovolt Corp.) The Spinco Analytrol is a calibrated recording photometer and automatic integrator and is recommended where larger numbers of procedures will be processed.

Paper strips: A suitable paper strip for the LKB apparatus has been found to be the Carl Schleicher and Schüll #2043B (120 Gm./m^2). A quantity of ready-for-use paper strips is provided for the LKB 3276BN paper electrophoresis apparatus; four of the 40 x 410 mm. strips may be placed in the cassette and run at the same time. The paper is also available in sheets of 580 x 580 mm. from which the required size can be cut. Cellulose acetate strips are available and give good uniformity and separation.[16, 17] (Consolidated Laboratories, Inc.)

Trays: These are used for staining and washing; a large pyrex baking dish may be utilized.

Spinco striper: This is used to apply serum samples to the paper strips. Its design insures that the measured quantity of serum is transferred evenly across the paper. It consists of two wires spaced 1mm. apart and coated with silicone for uniform surface tension.

Pipet: KMP or other ultramicro type, 10 lambdas.

Reagents

1. *Buffer solution:*   In all of our studies presented in this chapter, Veronal buffer has been used. This consists of a 0.1N sodium diethylbartiturate-0.02N diethylbarbituric acid solution of pH 8.6, ionic strength 0.1 in water. At this pH the serum proteins are negatively charged and will migrate toward the anode. To make 3 liters of buffer solution, dissolve 5.526 Gm. of diethylbarbituric acid (Veronal) and 30.927 Gm. of sodium barbital (sodium diethylbarbiturate) in 3 liters of water. Prepared buffer solution can be purchased.

It is possible to use the buffer solution for several runs if the quantities in both electrode vessels are poured together and mixed, one-third of it being discarded and replaced by a new buffer solution for each run. In doing this, the conditions remain essentially the same each time. At the same time the electrodes must be cleaned since the anode is found to collect varying amounts of precipitated salt after each run. If the direction of migration may be reversed, as in the Spinco cell, cleaning of the electrodes is unnecessary if the electrodes are each time reversed from that of the previous run.

2. *Dye solution:*

    0.01 per cent bromphenol blue

    5 per cent acetic acid (v/v)

    5 per cent $ZnSO_4 \cdot 7H_2O$ (w/v)

To prepare 2 liters, measure 100 ml. acetic acid, 100 Gm. $ZnSO_4 \cdot 7H_2O$ and 0.2 Gm. bromphenol blue. Dissolve in water and dilute to 2 liters.

Other dyes may be selected for particular purposes; e.g., sudan red, sudan black, or oil red O are used for identification of lipids and lipoid complexes.

The purity of the dye used, the dye-protein interaction, effect of protein denaturization, and degree of dye uptake are all important factors.[18]

Procedure—LKB Apparatus
(Fig. 47)

Preparation of Apparatus

1. Place the cassette, without lid, on a clear support, like a glass plate.

2. Place four strips of equal length in the cassette and fold downward between the vertical walls of either end of the cassette. Adjust the strips until they become parallel with each other and with the sides of the cassette and are *not touching each other.*

3. Fill each electrode vessel with about 900 ml. of Veronal solution, immerse the ends of the glass siphon in the solution and aspirate through the rubber tube until a buffer bridge is formed between the two electrode vessels. Press the rubber tube together with two fingers and hold the siphon so that the buffer solution can flow between the vessels until the equilibrium has ben obtained, *roughly 15 seconds.* The equilibration of buffer levels must be completed before each electro-chromatography run. Remove the glass siphon.

4. Connect the electrophoresis apparatus to a power supply outlet of 110 V. AC.

5. Before moistening the strips, it is best to place identifying data and position of the starting line on the strip in pencil. The position of the origin should be marked only by short lines or dots at the edge of the paper. A pencil line completely across the strip will give a *false reading* in the gamma-globulin area.

6. Place the cassette on top of the electrode vessels; the ends of the filter paper will be immersed in the buffer solution. Replace the lid of the cassette. The instrument is adjusted to a horizontal position with the aid of the spirit level. After about two hours the strips will be evenly moistened with the buffer solution.

7. The method of wetting the paper strips with the buffer solution affects the mobility of the serum. There is a possibility of a nonuniform distribution of electrolyte. It can be more evenly dispersed by allowing the wetted strips to equilibrate *for one hour* with the current *on* before applying the serum.

Application of Samples

The care and skill with which the application of the sample is carried out is one of the main factors necessary for a good analytical result. It is advantageous to have the starting line as thin and as smooth as

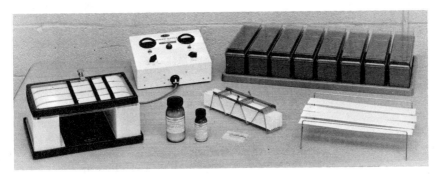

Fig. 47.—LKB paper electrophoresis equipment (Ivan Sorvall, Inc.)

possible. The serum, which does not have to be dialyzed, is applied to the paper strips as follows:

1.   Place a plexi-glass strip about 30 cm. long, 3 cm. wide and 3 mm. thick under the moist paper strips.

2.   Measure the amount of serum to be used (10 lambdas) with the ultramicro pipet and apply this to the Spinco striper. Place the sample on the previously marked starting place. The plexi-glass strip will serve as a support and *must be removed* as soon as the samples have been applied.

3.   When the paper strips have become displaced by the removal of the plexi-glass support, adjust them until they are again parallel with each other and with the longitudinal direction of the cassette.

4.   Turn on the power and adjust the instrument to a suitable current. *The analysis is now running.* Running time can be varied within rather wide limits; a separation can be obtained in *only four hours.* For a wider separation a longer run with a low current is advisable.

The current used should, in usual cases and in 4-8 hour runs, correspond to about 0.5 ma. for each 10 mm. width of filter paper. Four 40 mm. strips take a total current of 8 ma. For runs of longer duration, a lower current should be used; 0.25 ma./10 mm. for a 16 hour run, etc. It should be observed that the current will automatically increase during a run because of change in the resistance in the wet strip. For long-time runs it may be convenient to start with a current slightly lower than the average value. Our results have been obtained on these runs:

Starting current: 2.5 m/A (150) volts
Time: 16 hours (overnight)
Temperature: 8.7C (refrigerator)

Note: Temperature must be held constant since the mobilities of most ionic species increase by about two per cent for every degree rise in temperature.

5.   When the experiment has run for the desired length of time, shut off the current and *carefully* remove the lid of the cassette. No drops of water that adhere to the lower surface of the lid should fall on the paper strips.

Drying

1.   Remove the filter paper strips from the cassette and place them horizontally on a support so that the middle part of each strip (where the protein components are located) is freely suspended in air.

2.   Place this support with the strips in a drying oven at 110-120 C. *for 30 minutes.* It is important that the strips be *dried quickly.* By so doing diffusion of the edges of the individual zones can be kept to a minimum.

Variation in the amount of heat applied to the drying strips will cause varying degrees in denaturation of the proteins and will change the dye-binding properties of various protein components.[19-20] It has been demonstrated that after 30 minutes heating at 110-120 C., the dye uptake of albumin is about the same as for globulins.

Dyeing

1.   After drying, transfer the strips to the dye bath. They should be immersed *at least 5 hours* for it has been demonstrated that the uptake of dye by protein increases rapidly for the first 5 hours, then increases slowly up to 40 hours.[19] The relative amounts of dye taken up by the albumin and globulin fractions are constant from 5 to 16 hours. A large number of dyes have been examined and discussed by Griffiths.[21] The bromphenol blue reagent was preferred for general use.

Rinsing

1.   After dyeing, rinse the strips three times for 10 minutes at a time in 2 per cent acetic acid (v/v) *without agitation,* then rinse for 3 minutes in a bath of 2 per cent sodium acetate ($CH_3COONa \cdot 3H_2O$ w/v) in 10 per cent acetic acid (w/v). The last rinse impregnates the paper with sodium acetate. After the evaporation of acetic acid the dye remains as a blue sodium salt. Rinsing should remove all the dye mechanically trapped in the paper fiber but retain the dye bound to the protein. The rinsing procedure described removes most of this paper-bound dye.

2.   After being dried carefully on clean filter paper, the strips can be dried in air or in an oven for 10 to 15 minutes at 90-100 C. The paper strips are made translucent by dipping the strips into mineral oil, and drying them on clean filter paper to remove the excess oil. The strips are then ready for scanning.

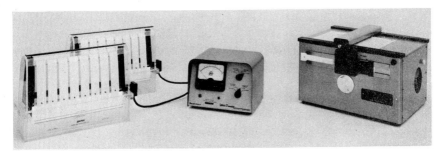

Fig. 48.—Spinco paper electrophoresis apparatus, with Duostat and Analytrol.

Procedure—Spinco Apparatus
(Fig. 48)

The operating instructions for the Spinco electrophoresis equipment are fully described in the operating manual supplied by the manufacturer. Directions are also available for the electrophoretic analysis of hemoglobins.

Evaluation

For quantitative analysis of the separated serum fractions in various areas of the filter paper, one of the following procedures may be followed.

1. *Measurement of extinction of the dye after elution:* If the components are well resolved and each spot can be definitely related to an electrophoretic species, the paper is cut into pieces, each containing only one component. The dye is extracted and the extract is filled up to a definite volume. The extinction value for each component extract is determined in a spectrophotometer and gives the relative concentration of the components in the sample.

If the components are badly resolved, the paper is cut in equally broad strips at right angles to the direction of migration. Each separate strip is extracted and the extinction is determined as mentioned above. The final determination of the component concentration will be obtained by constructing an electropherogram where the sum of optical densities of each area will represent the relative values of the area.

2. *Direct semi-automatic measurement:* In constructing an electropherogram from serum fractions present in various areas of filter paper, the optical densities at each interval will be plotted against the distance migrated. These points are then connected, thus completing the electropherogram. The instrument is zeroed on the paper in advance of the albumin and rechecked on the paper at the end of the gamma-globulin.

Vertical lines are drawn from the lowest point between two adjacent peaks to the base line. These lines define the area of each serum protein fraction. Since the areas are all related to each other and are determined by the optical densities and the distance measured in unit intervals, the only variable is that of optical density. Thus the areas of the various components are related to each other as the sum of the optical densities to each other.

For each serum fraction the optical densities are added, with the exception of the first and last reading in which one-half of the optical density of each is used. Total optical density for the pattern is obtained by adding the sums of the optical density for each protein component.[22] The relative percentage of each protein is in turn calculated:

$$\frac{\text{Sum of the optical densities assigned to the component}}{\text{Sum of the optical densities of the total}} \times 100$$

3. *Direct automatic measurement with the Analytrol:* The Analytrol (Spinco) consists of a photometer which measures and records light absorption in the paper strips and an integrator producing a saw-toothed pattern representing the area under the photometer curve immediately above. Detailed directions are provided by the manufacturer.

Calibration

In adapting paper electrophoresis to clinical use it is desirable to run comparative studies, when possible, between the paper and the classical Tiselius U-tube method. An example of this procedure is described by Köiw, Wallenius and Grönwall.[29] In our laboratories the Aminco-Stern Tiselius instrument was used as a basis of comparison and the method finally evolved was that closest in agreement with that machine. Many authors suggest the application of various numerical "factors" to bring the final results closer in agreement with the Tiselius technic. These factors are introduced to offset the numerous variables mentioned previously, and are not unlike factors frequently used by the undergraduate chemistry student to obtain desired results. We feel these add little more than confusion to the method; it is better to develop a method as reproducible and as similar to Tiselius as possible, reporting the absolute values that are obtained. Obviously the use of a filter paper introduces elements that affect the results not apparent in the U-tube method.

Normal Values

Normal values for the electrophoresis of human serum based on 20 normal adult persons:

TABLE 6.—ABSOLUTE

	Aminco Stern	Paper
Albumin	3.88 Gm./100 ml. ± 0.44	3.46 Gm./100 ml. ±0.37
a_1 globulin	0.37 Gm./100 ml. ± 0.09	0.37 Gm./100 ml. ± 0.11
a_2 globulin	0.68 Gm./100 ml. ± 0.12	0.66 Gm./100 ml. ± 0.14
β globulin	0.94 Gm./100 ml. ± 0.17	1.00 Gm./100 ml. ± 0.18
γ globulin	1.04 Gm./100 ml. ± 0.24	1.42 Gm./100 ml. ± 0.31

TABLE 7.—PERCENTAGES

	Aminco Stern	Paper
Albumin	56.1% ± 5.2	50.0% ± 5.4
a_1 globulin	5.4% ± 1.4	5.3% ± 1.6
a_2 globulin	9.9% ± 1.8	9.6% ± 2.1
β globulin	13.6% ± 2.5	14.5% ± 2.6
γ globulin	15.1% ± 3.3	20.6% ± 4.5

Note: Values by weight are based on total protein determination by the biuret method.

TABLE 8.—ELECTROPHORETIC ANALYSIS OF PLASMA PROTEINS IN CHILDREN AND ADULTS

Age	Sources of Data[23-28]	Number of Subjects	Albumin	a_1	a_2	β	θ	γ
Newborn	Longsworth	11	61.9	4.7	8.0	9.7	5.3	15.7
Newborn	Knapp & Routh	2	59.2	7.4	7.7	9.5	3.2	13.0
6-46 wks.	Knapp & Routh	11	61.7	6.7	12.9	11.5	3.8	3.3
2-4 yrs.	Lubschez	9	62.2	4.5	9.1	14.3	4.0	7.2
1-4 yrs.	Knapp & Routh	10	60.6	6.3	10.7	11.3	3.9	7.2
5-11 yrs.	Lubschez	21	57.3	5.1	9.7	11.9	5.7	10.4
5-11 yrs.	Knapp & Routh	17	56.6	6.2	9.8	12.0	5.7	9.7
13-17 yrs.	Knapp & Routh	14	60.6	5.0	9.7	10.9	5.0	8.7
Adult males:	Dole	15	60.3	4.6	7.2	12.1	5.1	11.0
	Deutsch	3	59.6	6.7	8.8	11.0	4.8	9.1
	Dryer	16	61.5	4.7	9.4	10.8	5.2	8.4

TABLE 9.—SERUM PROTEIN VALUES OF CORD BLOOD[30] (PERCENTAGES)

	Albumin	a_1	a_2	β	γ
Mean	41.3	7.1	11.6	12.6	27.4
Std. deviation	5.6	2.1	2.6	4.0	4.4

Note: The above values were determined by paper electrophoresis.

Studying the plasma proteins of 54 healthy children (ages birth to 17 years) by the Tiselius method, Knapp and Routh found the *percentage* of albumin decreased from infancy to mid-childhood and was lowest in children 5 to 11 years old; however, figures for the *absolute* concentration of albumin in Gm. per 100 ml. showed no significant decrease in albumin for this age group. The percentage and absolute concentration of α_2 globulin were highest in infancy and decreased gradually with age. Both the percentage and absolute concentration of gamma-globulin decreased from unusually high values in the newborn to unusually low values in infancy, and gradually reached the normal adult level in midchildhood—5-11 years of age.[23]

Discussion

The electrophoretic pattern obtained from serum is the result of many factors acting and interacting in a medium and reflects the physiologic state of the individual as a whole rather than any single pathologic condition. It promises to become one of the most valuable of clinical laboratory tests, particularly when combined with other methods of identification of the component fractions.

Electrophoretic analysis provides the most accurate value for the albumin to globulin ratio, and the best method for differentiation and quantitation of the various serum proteins and of hemoglobins. The development of paper electrochromatography places at the disposal of the pathologist and chemist a relatively simple and inexpensive method of obtaining information which formerly required extremely complicated and delicate apparatus; still further, it provides this information on 0.01 ml. of serum instead of the 20 ml. of serum previously needed.

In paper electrochromatography apparatus, the electric field is created by applying a voltage across two electrodes. When the space between the electrodes contains ionized particles in an aqueous buffer salt solution, the electric field will cause movement of the ions toward the electrodes. The movement of ions through the medium is governed by the frictional resistance of the medium. This resistance is related to the size and shape of the particles and the presence of a supporting substance, such as filter paper fibers which impede the movement of the particles.

Considerable ingenuity has been shown in devising methods of identification of the separated substances. These include study of their chemical properties or physical properties, fluorescence, nuclear reaction (e.g., radioactive tracers), emission spectra, migration rates and sequences, and biologic methods. Continual progress can be expected in the future in adapting electrochromatography to clinical use. An excellent review on interpretation of electropherograms is that of Owen[31] and—on principles and technics—the review of Peeters.[32]

REFERENCES

1. STRAIN, H. H., AND SATO, T. R.: *Anal. Chem. II 28:* 687, 1956.
2. RAYMOND, S.: Zone Electrophoresis, 2nd ed., New York, E. C. Apparatus Co., 1955.
3. KUNKEL, H. G., AND SLATER, R. J.: *Proc. Soc. Exper. Biol. & Med. 80:* 42, 1952.
4. ROTMAN, B., AND SPIEGELMAN, S.: *J. Bacteriol. 68:* 419, 1954.
5. TAMM, I., AND TYRELL, D. A.: *J. Immunol. 72:* 424, 1954.
6. FRANKLIN, E. C., HOLMAN, H. R., MÜLLER-EBERHARD, H. J., AND KUNKEL, H. G.: *J. Exper. Med. 105:* 425, 1957.
7. GERALD, P. S., AND DIAMOND, L. K.: *Blood 13:* 61, 1958.
8. GOLDBERG, C. A. J.: *Clin. Chem. 4:* 484, 1958.
9. ____: *Clin. Chem. 5:* 446, 1959.
10. STELOS, P., AND TALIAFERRO, W. H.: *Anal. Chem. 31:* 845, 1959.
11. FISHER, B.: *Am. J. Clin. Path. 23:* 246, 1953.
12. LEDERER, M.: An Introduction to Paper Electrophoresis and Related Methods. New York, Elsevier, 1957.
13. DURRUM, E. L.: *J. Am. Chem. Soc. 72:* 2943, 1950.
14. FLYNN, F. V., AND DE MAYO, P.: *Lancet 261:* 235, 1951.
15. LEVIN, B., AND OBERHOLZER, V. G.: *Am. J. Clin Path. 23:* 205, 1953.
16. KOHN, J.: *Clin. Chim. Acta 2:* 297, 1957.
17. ____: *Biochem. J. 65:* 9, 1957.
18. MARTIN, N. H.: Ciba Foundation Symposium on Paper Electrophoresis. Boston, Little, Brown & Co., 1956.
19. JENCKS, W. P., JETTON, M. R., AND DURRUM, E. L.: *Biochem. J. 60:* 205, 1955.
20. FRAGGLEN, G. T., AND MARTIN, N. H.: *Biochem. J. 57:* 626, 1954.
21. GRIFFITHS, L. L.: *J. Lab. & Clin. Med. 41:* 188, 1953.
22. MORRISON, D. B., AND SLOCUM, J.: *Am. J. Clin. Path. 25:* 1224, 1955.
23. KNAPP, E. L., AND ROUTH, J. L.: *Pediatrics 4:* 508, 1949.
24. LONGSWORTH, L. G., CURTIS, R. M., AND PEMBROKE, R. H.: *J. Clin. Invest. 24:* 46, 1945.
25. LUBSCHEZ, R.: *Pediatrics 2:* 570, 1948.
26. DOLE, V. P., AND BRAUN, E.: *J. Clin. Invest. 23:* 708, 1944.
27. DEUTSCH, H. F., AND GOODLOE, M. B.: *J. Biol. Chem. 161:* 1, 1945.
28. DRYER, R. L., PAUL, W. D., AND ROUTH, J. L.: *Proc. Soc. Exper. Biol. & Med. 66:* 552, 1947.
29. KÖIW, E., WALLENIUS, G., AND GRÖNWALL, A.: *Scandinav. J. Clin. & Lab. Inv. 4:* 47, 1952.
30. SOHAR, E., BOSSAK, E. T., WANG, C. I., AND ADLERSBERG, D.: *Science 123:* 461, 1956.
31. OWEN, J. A.: Advances in Clinical Chemistry, Vol. I, Sobotka, H., and Stewart, C. P., eds., New York, Academic Press, Inc., 1958, p. 237.
32. PEETERS, H.: Advances in Clinical Chemistry, Vol. II Sobotka, H., and Stewart, C. R., eds., New York, Academic Press, Inc., 1959, p. 2.

20

pH

BLOOD pH MEASUREMENT

Principle

The pH of venous or arterial blood is measured with a meter using a compensating type circuit (Metrohm Precision Compensator E 322) for maximum accuracy. A cathode ray tube is used as the zero indicator. Using the Metrohm capillary chain micro electrode (EA 518) designed by Sanz, a minimum of one drop of blood is required. Measurement is performed at body temperature.

Apparatus

Precision Compensator, E 322, Metrohm (Brinkmann Instruments, Inc.)
Micro blood electrode, EA 518, Metrohm
Thermostat, type F, Haake
Rubber vial stoppers, #68 MS Orange #3 (West. Co.)
Syringe, 2 ml.

Reagents

1. *Mercury*—reagent grade.

2. *Buffer and KCl solutions:* It is recommended that solutions for the Metrohm instrument be purchased from Brinkmann Instruments, Inc., as the buffers are standardized at 37 C. The Metrohm solutions supplied by Brinkmann for use in this procedure are:

Standard buffer, pH 6.975 at 37 C.
Standard buffer, pH 4.65 at 37 C.
Saturated gelatin-type KCl
Saturated KCl solution

Blood Collection

Analysis for pH should be scheduled in advance with the laboratory personnel responsible for carrying out the procedure. Blood is usually taken from a vein unless there is to be simultaneous determination of arterial oxygen saturation. Blood is drawn slowly into a 2 ml. syringe which has been rinsed previously with heparin; the syringe is capped immediately with a rubber vial stopper, being careful to exclude all air. The syringe and specimen are held in the clenched fist and taken immediately to the laboratory where the pH measurement is performed without delay. In this manner the specimen can be maintained close to body temperature, and pH changes within 10 minutes should be less than 0.01 pH units.[1] While there is probably no appreciable alteration in pH resulting from moderate temperature changes during this brief period, the final analysis is to be performed at 37 C. and it seems to us desirable to keep the specimen as close to that temperature as possible.

If any delay is anticipated in performing the analysis, the tip of the syringe should be placed in mercury immediately after collection and enough mercury drawn in to insure complete sealing. It is capped with a vial stopper and may be stored in ice water as long as 3 hours.[2]

When ready to measure the pH, shake the syringe to remix the blood. Remove the cap from the syringe, insert the tip of the plastic capillary deep into the blood, and draw a sample up into the micro capillary electrode. The pH of the blood sample is measured one minute later.

Capillary blood specimens are collected in the manner developed by Lilienthal and Riley.[3, 4] This technic is also described in detail by Gambino.[2] The capillary bed of the ear or finger is arterialized with heat—a light bulb held close to the ear is sufficient, or the finger may be immersed in 40 to 45 C. water for 5 minutes. After cleaning and drying the puncture site, the capillary bed is incised with a No. 11 Bard-Parker scalpel blade to a depth of 5 to 7 mm. Blood is permitted to flow freely from the incision and the drops of blood are all collected in a rubber cap attached to the tip of a tightly-fitting 2 ml. syringe. Gambino recommends fashioning this rubber cap from the stopper of a 10 ml. Vacutainer tube (Becton-Dickinson and Co.). The dead space within the syringe is filled with 1 per cent ammonium heparinate. The blood which drops into the rubber cup is slowly drawn into the syringe. After sufficient blood has been collected, the rubber cup is removed and mercury is drawn into the syringe for sealing and mixing. The syringe is capped with a rubber vial stopper and the procedure carried out as with venous blood.

Other technics of collecting venous and capillary blood are described in the medical literature.[5-12]

Procedure

1.   Connect the Haake thermostat to the water supply, adjust water flow to one-half liter per minute.

2.   Turn the thermostat's master switch on. The temperature is regulated to exactly 37 C. (This is done by means of the contact thermometer corrected with a precision thermometer.)

3.   Turn on the E 322 compensator by tripping the line switch (8).

4.   Remove rubber stopper from the reference electrode and check to see if completely filled with saturated KCl.

5.   Allow both the thermostat and compensator to warm up for 20 minutes.

6.   Put function switch (1) on *CALIBRATE*.

7.   With measuring key (9) in 0 position, balance cathode ray indicator (7) with potentiometer for zero adjustment (11). *This is labeled 0 on the instrument.*

8.   Push measuring key upwards. If the strips of the cathode ray indicator are not at the same level, correct with calibrating potentiometer (10). *This is labeled E on the instrument.*

9.   Put buffer in capillary electrode and immerse both electrodes in saturated gelatine-type KCl. *The buffer and later the sample should form a complete column of liquid in the capillary electrode and be free of bubbles.*

10.   Turn function switch to pH 37 C.

11.   The pH value of the buffer is attained with manipulations of the step switch (2) and the fine compensator (3).

12.   Actuate measuring key, first on position of low sensitivity (downward position), then on high sensitivity (upward position), and compensation is performed with compensating voltage calibrator (5).

13.   Now the apparatus is calibrated to the measuring chain in use and the compensator (5) must not be moved during subsequent measurements.

14.   Remove the electrodes from the saturated KCl, thoroughly rinse with distilled water and wipe off with filter paper.

15.   The blood to be measured is drawn into the capillary electrode and compensation performed by means of the measuring key (9) and compensating potentiometer (3).

16.   The measured pH value is indicated by the position of step switch (2) and fine compensator (3).

17.   The capillary electrode is rinsed with saline between samples.

18.   Recheck the pH calibration with the buffer of pH 6.975.

19.   When finished, the capillary electrode is thoroughly rinsed with

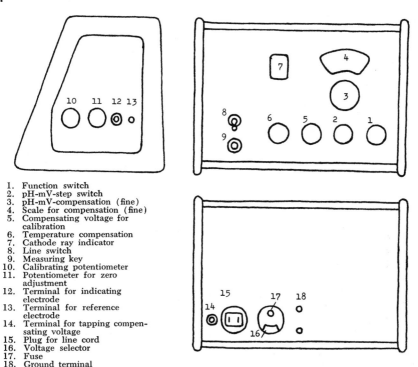

1. Function switch
2. pH-mV-step switch
3. pH-mV-compensation (fine)
4. Scale for compensation (fine)
5. Compensating voltage for calibration
6. Temperature compensation
7. Cathode ray indicator
8. Line switch
9. Measuring key
10. Calibrating potentiometer
11. Potentiometer for zero adjustment
12. Terminal for indicating electrode
13. Terminal for reference electrode
14. Terminal for tapping compensating voltage
15. Plug for line cord
16. Voltage selector
17. Fuse
18. Ground terminal

Fig. 49.—Metrohm Precision Compensator E 322.

saline and then with distilled water. The electrode is filled with acetate buffer or with water and the tip left immersed in either buffer or water solution.

The reference electrode is stored in saturated KCl solution and the filling nipple is closed with the rubber stopper.

20. The pH meter and thermostat are then turned off.

Note: Liquid must be kept in the capillary electrode when the thermostat is in operation to prevent drying out of the gel zone.

Normal Values

pH 7.37 to 7.42 (arterial blood)

Discussion

In both compensated acidosis and alkalosis the plasma pH remains within the normal range. In severe metabolic and respiratory acidosis the pH falls below 7.30 and in severe metabolic and respiratory alkalosis the pH rises above 7.50.

In alkalosis the plasma pH tends to rise. In metabolic alkalosis the plasma bicarbonate is raised; this may be due to excessive alkali ingestion or to greater loss of chloride relative to sodium. This condition also occurs with potassium depletion. With respiratory alkalosis the plasma bicarbonate is reduced as a result of hyperventilation.

The plasma pH tends to fall with acidosis. In metabolic acidosis the plasma bicarbonate is reduced; this condition may be brought on by starvation, ammonium chloride ingestion, diabetes mellitus, severe diarrhea, renal failure and renal tubular disease. With respiratory acidosis resulting from emphysema, pneumonia, pulmonary congestion, lung destruction, or morphine, the plasma bicarbonate is raised.

In health, the pH of arterial blood varies from about 7.3 to 7.5. This range of pH is only 0.2, but it should be kept in mind that the concentration of H^+ is more than 50 per cent greater at one extreme of this range than at the other. The extreme range of pH which is still compatible with life is 6.95 to 7.80.

Other instruments for pH measurement, including refinements of the Metrohm apparatus, are discussed in the chapter on Special Equipment.

REFERENCES

1. GAMBINO, S. R.: *Am. J. Clin. Path. 32:* 270, 1959.
2. _____: *Am. J. Clin. Path. 35:* 175, 1961.
3. LILIENTHAL, J. L., JR., AND RILEY, R. L.: *J. Clin. Invest. 23:* 904, 1944.
4. _____: *J. Lab. & Clin. Med. 31:* 999, 1946.
5. SHOCK, N. W., AND HASTINGS, A. B.: *Proc. Soc. Exper. Biol. & Med. 26:* 780, 1929.
6. _____: *J. Biol. Chem. 104:* 565, 1934.
7. NATELSON, S.: Microtechniques of Clinical Chemistry for the Routine Laboratory. Springfield, Ill., Charles C Thomas, 1957.
8. SANZ, M. C.: *Clin. Chem. 3:* 406, 1957.
9. ASTRUP, P.: Astrum Micro Equipment Bulletin No. 21917A. Copenhagen, Radiometer Co., 1960.
10. GAMBINO, S. R.: *Am. J. Clin. Path. 32:* 285, 1959.
11. _____: Workshop on Microchemistry—Technique Manual. Chicago, Ill., American Soc. Clin. Pathol., 1960.
12. BROOKS, D., AND WYNN, V.: *Lancet 1:* 227, 1959.
13. Operating Instructions for E 322 Compensator, Haake Thermostat Type "F" and Capillary Electrode EA 518. Herisau, Switzerland, Scientific Instruments, Metrohm Ltd., 1959.

21

Salicylates

TRINDER'S METHOD

Principle

The proteins in an unknown serum are precipitated in acid solution by mercuric chloride. Ferric ion reacts with salicylic acid and forms a purple color. The purple color developed is compared with a standard salicylate solution treated similarly.[1]

Apparatus

Pipets, KMP or other ultramicro type, 250 lambdas (2)
Pipet, KMP or other ultramicro type, 25 lambdas

Reagents

1. *Trinder's reagent:* Transfer 4.0 Gm. ferric nitrate ($[Fe(NO_3)_3 \cdot 9H_2O]$) and 4.0 Gm. mercuric chloride ($HgCl_2$) into a 100 ml. volumetric flask. Add 12 ml. of 1 N hydrochloric acid, dissolve in water and dilute to the mark. Filter. This solution is stable indefinitely.

2. *Standard (25 mg./100 ml. salicylic acid):* Dissolve 0.29 Gm. sodium salicylate in water and dilute to 1 liter or dissolve 0.25 Gm. salicylic acid in water and dilute to 1 liter.

Procedure

1. Transfer 250 lambdas of distilled water into each of three 1 ml. micro centrifuge tubes labeled *test*, *standard*, and *reagent blank*.

2. Add 25 lambdas distilled water to the *reagent blank* tube, 25 lambdas of serum to the tube marked *test*, and 25 lambdas salicylate standard to the tube for *standard*. Mix.

3. To each tube add 250 lambdas of Trinder's reagent, mix, and let stand for 5 minutes.

4. **Centrifuge for an additional five minutes.**

5. **Transfer the clear supernatants into ultramicro cuvets and read the optical density against water at 540 mμ.**

Calculation

$$\frac{\text{mg. per 100 ml. salicylic acid in standard}}{(\text{O.D. standard minus O.D. blank})} \times (\text{O.D. test minus O.D. blank}) = \frac{\text{mg. per 100 ml. salicylate in unknown}}{}$$

ALTERNATE METHOD

Principle

This method also utilizes the color reaction between salicylate and iron. It is a simple technic which has given satisfactory results for clinical purposes.[2-4]

Apparatus

Pipets, KMP or other ultramicro type, 250 lambdas (2)
Pipet, KMP or other ultramicro type, 25 lambdas

Reagents

1. *Ferric nitrate, 1.0 per cent w/v:* Solvent is 0.07 N nitric acid. Dissolve 10.0 Gm. ferric nitrate [Fe(NO$_3$)$_3$·9H$_2$O] in 0.07 N nitric acid and dilute to 1 liter.

2. *Nitric acid, 0.07 N:* Dilute 4.69 ml. of H$_2$NO$_3$ (specific gravity 1.42, 70.7 per cent) to 1 liter with water.

3. *Salicylate standard, 50 mg./100 ml.:* Dissolve 0.580 Gm. sodium salicylate in water and dilute to 1 liter, or dissolve 0.500 Gm. salicylic acid in water and dilute to 1 liter.

Procedure

1. **Transfer 250 lambdas of distilled water into each of four 1 ml. micro centrifuge tubes labeled *test*, *standard*, *serum blank*, and *reagent blank*.**

2. **Add 25 lambdas of serum to the tubes marked *test* and *serum blank*; add 25 lambdas of salicylate standard to the tube marked *standard* and 25 lambdas of distilled water to the tube marked *reagent blank*.**

3. **Add 250 lambdas of ferric nitrate solution to the tubes marked** *test, standard,* **and** *reagent blank.* **Mix.**

4. **Add 250 lambdas of 0.07 N nitric acid to the tube marked** *serum blank,* **mix, and let stand for 5 minutes.**

5. **Read in Beckman DU spectrophotometer at 540 mμ.**

Calculation

$$\frac{\text{mg./100 ml. salicylate in standard}}{\text{O.D standard—O.D. reagent blank}} \times (\text{O.D. unknown—O.D. serum blank}) = \frac{\text{mg./100 ml. salicylate in unknown}}{}$$

Note: Aspirin is an acetylated form of salicylic acid and is converted to free salicylic acid in the body. This method measures the free salicylic acid. The amount of color formed is in direct proportion to the quantity of salicylate present.[2-4] This method is accurate within ± 3 per cent and has good reproducibility.

Normal Values

Salicylates are not normally present in the blood. As most of the determinations are performed on known or suspected cases of poisoning, more meaningful interpretations of their significance can be made if the time of ingestion of the salicylate can be ascertained. Done[5] has pointed out the value of calculating the theoretical initial salicylate level or estimating it through the use of a nomogram. The nomogram relates serum salicylate concentration and the expected severity of intoxication at varying intervals following the ingestion of a single dose of salicylate.

Estimating Severity of Salicylate Intoxication[*]
On Basis of Initial Salicylate Level (S_I)
$$\log S_I = \log S_S + .015\ T$$

S_I (mg./100 ml.)	Effect
50	asymptomatic
50-80	mild
80-100	moderate
110	severe
160	usually fatal

S_I = initial level of salicylate; S_S = serum salicylate in mg./100 ml.; T = time in hours.

* From work of A. K. Done.[5]

Discussion

Salicylates, in various forms, are probably the most widely used medicine today. It was estimated in 1944 that the average production of acetylsalicylic acid in the United States amounted to over 6 million pounds a year.[6] Natural salicylates, existing largely as salicin and methyl salicylate, have been used since the time of Hippocrates; today they have been largely replaced by sodium salicylate, methyl salicylate, phenyl salicylate, acetyl salicylic acid, and para-aminosalicylic acid.

The potential toxicity of salicylates is now widely recognized, although the protean manifestations have yet to be completely explained. The use of salicylates has been found to increase the frequency of bleeding in peptic ulcer patients; it appears that the effect is one of augmenting gastric acidity rather than any direct depression of prothrombin activity.[7, 8] Fever, rash, nausea, emesis, arthralgia and neuralgia have been encountered with the use of para-aminosalicylic acid.[9] Hypokalemia has also been observed.[10, 11]

The problem of accidental and therapeutic salicylate intoxication in children has been very completely described by Riley and Worley.[12] These authors, reviewing 42 cases of salicylate intoxication, found the majority of cases of accidental poisoning occurring in children 2-4 years old, while most of the intoxication during therapy was seen in infants. They attribute most of the difficulties: overdosage, decreased renal excretion of salicylates due to renal immaturity, and prerenal azotemia from associated dehydration. The estimation of plasma salicylates is important in following the progress of a case, although as these and other authors have pointed out, severe symptoms can be present even when low concentrations of salicylate are present in the plasma.

Normal serum may contain substances which give a salicylate type reaction as high as 2 mg./100 ml.; acetoacetic acid is believed to account for much of this reaction.[13]

REFERENCES

1. TRINDER, P.: *Biochem. J. 57:* 301, 1954.
2. BRODIE, B. B., UNDENFRIEND, S., AND CORBUN, A. F.: *The determination of salicylic acid in plasma. J. Pharmacol. & Exper. Therap. 80:* 114, 1944.
3. KELLER, W. J.: *Am. J. Clin. Path. 17:* 145, 1947.
4. TARNSKY, A. L., AND BREWS, A. L.: *J. Clin. Path. 3:* 289, 1950.
5. DONE, A. K.: *Pediatrics 26:* 800, 1960.
6. GROSS, M., AND GREENBERG, L. A.: The Salicylates. A Critical Biographic Review. New Haven, Hillhouse Press, 1948.
7. KELLY, J. J., JR.: *Am. J. M. Sc. 232:* 119, 1956.
8. NORVIIT, L., AND CARSTENSEN, B.: *Am. Rev. Tuberc. 67:* 258, 1953.
9. KORST, D. H.: *Ann. Int. Med. 40:* 1011, 1954.
10. CAYLEY, F. E., DE W.: *Lancet 1:* 447, 1950.

11. McIntyre, P. A.: *Bull. Johns Hopkins Hosp. 92:* 210, 1953.
12. Riley, H. D., and Worley, L.: *Pediatrics 18:* 578, 1956.
13. Meites, S., and Faulkner, W. R.: Manual of Practical Micro and General Procedures in Clinical Chemistry, Springfield, Ill., Charles C Thomas, 1962.

Additional References:
Volterra, M., and Jacobs, M. D.: *J. Lab. & Clin. Med. 32:* 1282, 1947.
MacDonald, R. P., Ploompuu, J., and Knights, E. M., Jr.: *Pediatrics 20:* 515, 1957.

22

Sodium and Potassium

The development of practical flame photometry has been described as one of the most important advances in modern clinical chemistry. The elements to be analyzed are excited by a flame and the spectral lines of these elements are isolated by suitable filters. The lines are focused on a photocell that converts this light energy to electrical energy which may be quantitated by use of a galvanometer.

The procedures described here are for the double photocell technic of analysis (Baird-Atomic KY-1, Baird Flame Photometer, Advanced Flame Photometer) and the single photocell method (Coleman). These instruments are described in the section on special equipment.

DOUBLE PHOTOCELL METHOD:
1) Advanced Flame Photometer

General Points

Always turn the water pump on before lighting the burner. Calibration is performed with two knobs, the coarse on the left, the fine on the right. Calibrate on "M" standard only. Always center the meter when reading; the solution should be at the same level in the funnel each time. It is best to make a mark one-quarter inch from the funnel apex. Whenever you pour in the "M" standard, set MEASURE at 500, and *do not* adjust MEASURE further. Use CALIBRATE instead to center the meter. To read unknowns or other standards, always use MEASURE—do not use CALIBRATE. For the highest accuracy always calibrate "M" standard after unknowns or other standard. Do not look for a straight line between standards. (If you have been used to a straight line over the entire serum range, you have been straightening out a curve for simplicity. No flame signal is a straight line if your standards are exact.) This instrument has practically no drift, but the alternating technic—recalibrating at the midpoint between unknowns—is recommended. The stylet wire should be passed through the atomizer after each serum run. Knobs should be turned slowly.

Apparatus

Flame photometer, advanced
Pipets, KMP or other ultramicro type, 100 lambdas
Pipets, KMP or other ultramicro type, 50 lambdas
Volumetric flasks, glass stoppered, 10 and 5 ml.
Stylets (Clay-Adams A-2451)

Reagents

1. Only one set of standards is necessary to cover the normal serum range. Each standard contains both Na and K. The series is based on 1:100 dilution of serum. Three standards are useful. Five or seven will more accurately determine the shape of the curve.

2. To make a series of three, each should contain:

Standard Designation	Na	K	Li
"L"	1.2 mEq./L. and	0.03 mEq./L. and	300 ppm
"M"	1.4 mEq./L. and	0.05 mEq./L. and	300 ppm
"H"	1.6 mEq./L. and	0.07 mEq./L. and	300 ppm

3. Do not confuse quantities and concentrations. To keep these straight when mixing solutions, always use this equation:

$$\frac{\text{Final concentration desired}}{\text{Starting concentration}} = \frac{\text{ml. of starting concentration}}{\text{ml. of volumetric flask}}$$

4. For example, using advanced concentrated solutions, to make up "M" standard in a 500 ml. flask:

Put in 14 ml. of 500 mEq./L. Na, $\quad \dfrac{1.4}{50} = \dfrac{x}{500} \quad x = 14$ ml.

and 1.25 ml. of 20 mEq./L. K, $\quad \dfrac{0.05}{20} = \dfrac{y}{500} \quad y = 1.25$ ml

and 30 ml. of 500 ppm Li $\quad \dfrac{300}{5000} = \dfrac{z}{500} \quad z = 30$ ml.

QS to volume with distilled water.

Procedure

Preparation of unknown samples: Transfer 100 lambdas of serum to a test tube or flask graduated at 10 ml. Dilute to 10 ml. mark with solution containing 303 ppm lithium. This gives a final lithium concentration of 300 ppm, and saves the extra pipetting step. Both Na and K determinations can be run from this flask.

Directions for use of advanced flame photometer:

1. Turn on pump.
2. Turn on air supply.
3. Turn on gas, remove chimney and light the flame.
4. Turn Selector Switch to Na or K position.

Allow machine to warm up 20-30 minutes. While machine is warming up, run several funnels of "M" Standard through.

5. Set *Measure* at 500 and pour M Standard.
6. Adjust needle to center position with *Calibration* controls.
7. Pour H Standard, return needle to center with *Measure* and record reading on dial.
8. Repeat steps 5 and 6.
9. Pour L Standard, center needle with *Measure* and record reading on dial.
10. Repeat steps 5 through 9 until readings are consistent.
11. When readings are consistent, plot these three points on a graph with dial readings vs. mEq./L. The resultant graph should not be a straight line.
12. Pour M standard; center needle with *Calibrate*.
13. Pour unknown; center needle with *Measure* and record reading.
14. Repeat steps 12 and 13 until all unknowns are read and recorded.
15. Compare readings to graph and determine mEq./L.'s for unknowns.
16. If all unknowns are satisfactory, pour distilled water through funnel.
17. Turn machine off as follows:
    a. Selector switch OFF
    b. Gas off
    c. Air off
    d. Pump off

DOUBLE PHOTOCELL METHOD:
2) Baird-Atomic Model KY-1

General Points

This instrument should be on electrically for 24 hours prior to operation;

it is best to leave it on permanently. It should not be placed in either direct or reflected sunlight, and for accurate results the surrounding illumination should be constant. The flame should be lit 15 minutes prior to standardizing the instrument, and distilled water should be run through the funnel. This establishes a proper operating temperature in the glassware. Always standardize before operating. The manufacturer recommends placing an inverted 500 ml. plastic bottle in the funnel before and after use to keep the atomizer and chamber at constant temperature and ready for immediate readings.

Apparatus

Flame Photometer, Baird-Atomic, Inc., Model KY-1
Pipets, KMP or other ultramicro type, 50 lambdas
Pipets, KMP or other ultramicro type, 500 lambdas
Volumetric flasks, 10 ml.

Reagents

Working standard solutions (prepare from Baird-Atomic concentrated solutions.) Store in polyethylene bottles.

Procedure

1. **Turn on the air supply and adjust it to 6 psi. Be sure red pilot light is on.**
2. **Hold lighted match at chimney rim and turn on gas.**
3. **If gas does not ignite, reduce air pressure and repeat. After gas ignites, return air pressure to 6 psi.**
4. **Run distilled water through funnel for 10-15 minutes.**
5. **Standardize as follows for serum samples:**
   a) **The meter should read within 4.8 and 5.2 on the lower scale (with no solution in funnel). If not, use the K ZERO control to correct K reading (on lower scale) and Na ZERO to correct the Na reading to 139-141 on the upper scale.**
   b) **Pour 140/5 standard into the funnel. Set selector switch to K. Adjust K CENTER to read 5 on lower scale. Turn switch to Na. Adjust Na CENTER to read 140 on upper scale. After reading, always remove liquid from funnel.**
   c) **Pour 160/9 standard into the funnel. Wait 30 seconds. Set switch to K. Adjust K RANGE to read 9 on lower scale. Turn switch to Na. Adjust Na RANGE to read 160 on upper scale.**
   d) **Repeat steps b) and c) until readings reproduce within one**

division. **Pour 120/1 into funnel. K should read 1 and Na 120 to within one division.**

e) **Pour the properly diluted sample into the funnel. (A 50-lambda sample is added to 500 lambdas of 5000 ppm Li and diluted with distilled water to a total of 10 ml. in a volumetric flask.) With the selector switch at K, the lower scale reading gives the concentration of potassium in mEq./L. in the original undiluted sample. With the selector switch at Na, the upper scale reading gives the concentration of sodium in mEq./L. in the original undiluted sample.**

DOUBLE PHOTOCELL METHOD:
3) Baird Flame Photometer

Flame photometer, Baird
Pipet, KMP or other ultramicro type, 50 lambdas
Pipet, KMP or other ultramicro type, 100 lambdas
Test tubes, Klett, grad. at 5 and 10 ml.
Bottles, polyethylene, screw cap, cap. 32 oz.
Washing bottles, polyethylene, squeeze type, cap. 8 oz.

Reagents

It is recommended that stock standard solutions be purchased from Baird Associates. The difficulty of avoiding even slight contamination in preparation and of obtaining constant weights of the salts makes laboratory preparation impractical. The solutions supplied by Baird contain the following cation concentrations:

Li (LiNO$_3$)	5000 ppm
K (KCl)	20 mEq./L.
Na (NaCl)	50 mEq./L.

In preparing the working standards and the Li diluting solution, clean all glassware to be used with a chromic acid cleaning solution and rinse several times with distilled water.

1. *Lithium diluting solution:* Dilute 40 ml. of stock solution (5000 ppm) to 2 L. with distilled water. Take precautions to avoid contamination from finger and other sources. Store in polyethylene or Pyrex bottle.

2. *Potassium working standard solution:** Dilute the following volumes of

---

* Avoid contamination by taking the precautions for reagents mentioned and store in polyethylene bottles.

stock potassium standard solutions with lithium diluting solution:

    7 ml. 500 ml. (equivalent to 7 mEq./L.)

    5 ml. to 500 ml. (equivalent to 5 mEq./L.)

    3 ml. to 500 ml. (equivalent to 3 mEq./L.)

    3. *Sodium working standard solution:** Dilute the following volumes of stock sodium standard solutions with lithium diluting solution:

    8 ml. to 500 ml. (equivalent to 160 mEq./L.)

    7 ml. to 500 ml. (equivalent to 140 mEq./L.)

    6 ml. to 500 ml. (equivalent to 120 mEq./L.)

Working standard solutions are conveniently dispensed into the atomizer from polyethylene squeeze type wash bottles. One bottle may also be used for distilled water, another for removing excess solution from the atomizer funnel after a reading has been taken. The latter should have the inside tubing cut off just below the bottle cap.

Procedure

Preparation of sodium sample: Transfer 50 lambdas of serum to a test tube graduated at 5 and 10 ml. containing about 5 ml. of lithium solution and rinse the pipet by drawing in and expelling mixture several times. Dilute to 10 ml. mark with Li diluting solution. Stopper with specially cleaned stopper and mix thoroughly. (25 lambdas of serum and 5 ml. of Li solution may be used if it is necessary to reduce the quantity of serum used.)

Preparation of potassium sample: Transfer 100 lambdas of serum to a test tube graduated at 5 and 10 ml. Add 2 or 3 ml. of Li solution and rinse pipet by drawing in and expelling mixture several times. Dilute to 5 ml. mark with Li solution. Stopper with specially cleaned stopper and mix thoroughly. (See *Discussion* for alternate dilutions using less seurm, page 187.)

Directions for use of flame photometer.

1. Plug in galvanometer and allow to warm up 15-20 minutes.

2. Adjust air pressure to 10 lbs. *Caution:* Air must be turned on before gas.

3. Turn gas on slowly while holding lighted match over the top of the burner chimney. When burner lights, adjust flame so that no yellow color appears and flame is about 2 inches from top of chimney. Small cones of blue flame should appear just above the burner grid.

4. Set middle switch of photometer on *Direct Method.* Set *Balance*

---

    * Avoid contamination by taking the precautions for reagents mentioned and store in polyethylene bottles.

dial on 700 and filter dial (top of instrument) on *K*. Adjust galvanometer to zero by means of coarse adjustment (lever on top of case) and fine adjustment (knob on side of case). The dial cross hair should bisect the zero on the dial.

5.   Set middle switch of photometer on *Internal Standard*. Pour the highest standard (7 mEq./L. of K) into atomizer funnel. Adjust galvanometer to zero by means of the sensitivity dial. The point may be marked on the dial for approximate reference with a red wax pencil.

6.   After this standard has completely run through the atomizer (galvanometer cross hair will shift away from zero), change middle switch of photometer back to *Direct* and re-check the zero setting on the galvanometer.

7.   Readjust galvanometer if necessary to bring it to zero. If galvanometer is readjusted, repeat steps 5 and 6 until galvanometer reads zero in both cases.

8.   Pour middle standard (5 mEq./L. of K) into atomizer funnel switch middle dial to *Internal Standard* and adjust balance dial until the cross hair of the galvanometer bisects zero. Read scale on balance dial. It should read 500 ± 004. If it fails to do this, repeat steps 5-8. If it does read zero, proceed to step 9.

9.   After atomizer funnel has been cleared of the solution, pour the low standard (3 mEq./L.) into the funnel and adjust galvanometer to zero with the balance dial. It should read 300 ± 004. If not, re-check the other standards. If it does, proceed with step 10. (It may help when re-checking to move the balance dial so that the galvanometer cross hair moves away from zero, and then return the cross hair to zero with the balance dial.)

10.   After the instrument has been calibrated, run the unknown specimens through by adjusting the cross hair to zero with the balance dial and reading mEq. of patassium directly from the balance scale. Be sure to allow sufficient time for the atomizer to empty one sample before pouring in the next.

11.   After finishing the potassium determination, set the filter dial on *Na*, the *Balance* dial on 800 for the 160 mEq./L. standard and proceed as for K. The other two standards are equivalent to 140 and 120 mEq./L. respectively and the balance scale should read 700 and 600 ± 004 for these standards. No readjustment of the burner is necessary when switching dials from *K* to *Na*.

12.   After completing the test, run distilled water through the atomizer twice and shut off the gas followed by the air. (Reverse of lighting burner.)

Calculations

Balance Dial Reading $\times$ F = mEq./L.

A. *Potassium:*

Dilution	Factor
1:80	3.20
1:60	2.40
1:66.7	2.67
1:50	2.00

Note: Read balance dial for potassium as two decimal places, i.e. 3.50.

B. *Sodium:*

Dilution	Factor
1:200	2.0

Note: Read balance dial for sodium as one decimal place, i.e. 60.0.

C. mEq./L. Na $\times$ 2.3 = mg. per 100 ml.

mEq./L. K $\times$ 3.91 = mg. per 100 ml.

SINGLE PHOTOCELL METHOD: COLEMAN

Apparatus

Flame photometer, Coleman model 21
Galv-O-Meter, Coleman model 22
Pipets, KMP or other ultramicro type, 20 lambdas
Volumetric flasks, 2 ml.
Plastic micro cups, Coleman, 2 ml.
Bottles, polyethylene, screw cap, cap. 32 oz.
Wash bottles, polyethylene, squeeze type, 8 oz.

Reagents

1. *Stock standards:*

Standard Reagent A (100 mEq./L. Sodium). Weigh 5.845 Gm. of desiccated reagent grade NaCl, dissolve in water and *quantitatively* transfer into 1000 ml. volumetric flask. Fill to the mark with water and mix well. Store only in Pyrex or polyethylene bottles.

Standard reagent B (5 mEq./L. Potassium). Weigh 0.3728 Gm. of desiccated reagent grade KCl, dissolve in water and *quantitatively* transfer into a 1000 ml. volumetric flask. Fill to the mark with water and mix well. Store only in Pyrex or polyethylene bottles.

1 per cent Sterox SE Stock Solution. Pipet 5 ml. of Sterox into a 500 ml. volumetric flask, fill to the mark with water, mix well, and store only in Pyrex or polyethylene bottles.

0.02 per cent Sterox SE. Pipet 10 ml. of 1 per cent Sterox into a 500 ml. volumetric flask, fill to the mark and mix well.

2. *Working standards:*

*Sodium and potassium working standards** 10 ml. of 1 per cent Sterox are added to the following volumes of standard reagent A and standard reagent B and each solution made to a final volume of 500 ml. with water.

1 per cent sterox (ml.)	*Standard Reagent A* (ml.)	*Standard Reagent B* (ml.)	*Na* (mEq./L.)	*K* (mEq./L.)
10	8	8	160	8
10	7	7	140	7
10	6	5	120	5
10	5	2	100	2

Procedure

Preparation of sodium and potassium samples: Any volume of sample may be taken for analysis; however, it must be diluted 100-fold. Transfer 20 lambdas of serum to a 2 ml. volumetric flask containing approximately 1 ml. of water, rinsing the pipet several times. Add 1 drop of 1 per cent Sterox, make to volume with water, and mix by inversion. Transfer these along with the working standards to 2 ml. plastic micro cups shortly before use.

Directions for use of flame photometer: The technic as here described is for the Coleman Model 21 flame photometer with the Coleman Model 22 Galv-O-Meter operated as the indicating galvanometer. The Coleman autoflow system may be used. Experience will determine the volume of diluted sample which will be required for making a reading.

1.   Plug cables from Model 22 Galv-O-Meter and from flame attachment into a 120 V outlet. Allow instruments to warm up for 15 minutes.

2.   Keep working cell of Galv-O-Meter disconnected by turning STD control full counterclockwise. This makes the BAL knob position immaterial.

---

* Based on a 1:100 dilution of serum.

3. Disconnect Galv-O-Meter from flame unit to check 0 reading (black scale) by unplugging the connecting wire on the Galv-O-Meter end. Then make a rough zero setting with the adjusting lever and follow with a fine 0 setting by adjusting the sliding scale panel. Reinsert the connecting wire.

4. Turn shutoff valve ON.

5. Turn on gas full and light burner.

6. Bring oxygen pressure up to 13 lb./in.^{2} slowly.

7. Place Na filter in slot, the symbol toward the operator.

8. Set the GALV course control completely counterclockwise and the GALV fine control about midway clockwise.

9. Steadiness control on 10.

10. Close door on flame unit and zero the Galv-O-Meter by using the BLK course and BLK fine controls on the flame photometer. No solution is used for the zero setting.

11. Set the transmission scale at 80 while atomizing the standard of highest concentration by using the GALV controls on the Galv-O-Meter.

12. Recheck zero setting and then recheck the 80 reading with more standard.

13. Read the remaining standards and the samples. Use 0.02 per cent Sterox for flushing the capillary. Recheck the 80 setting with the standard at regular intervals and at the end of the determination.

14. Flush the system with 0.02 per cent Sterox.

15. Insert the K filter in the slot. The symbol toward the operator.

16. Set the GALV course control about one-quarter turn from counter-clockwise and the GALV fine control one-half turn from counterclockwise.

17. Steadiness control on 10.

18. Repeat steps 10 to 14.

19. In turning the instrument off, first turn off oxygen and then turn off gas without delay.

20. Plot the values obtained for the standards on linear paper, plotting per cent transmission scale readings vs. concentration of Na or K in mEq./L. of serum. Galv-O-Meter readings of samples are then converted to corresponding Na or K concentrations. The curve for K is linear, while the curve for Na is not.

Normal Values

Adults and Children

Na: 135-150 mEq./L.   K: 3.5-5.6 mEq./L.

See also the discussion of full-term and premature infants.

The normal value ranges for 90 per cent of children are presented by Gyllenswärd and Josephson:[16]

TABLE 10.

Normal Limits for Serum Sodium, Potassium, and Chloride

	Limits	Newborn	3 mo.	6 mo.	9 mo.	12 mo.	3-6 yr.
Na	Upper	154.6	150.7	145.7	148.4	157.2	144.2
	Lower	122.0	117.5	119.9	116.6	110.8	115.7
K	Upper	5.46	6.48	6.25	6.11	5.90	5.69
	Lower	3.84	3.99	3.84	3.95	3.75	2.69
Cl	Upper	109.2	148.7	136.7	135.8	137.4	121.0
	Lower	106.2	78.4	80.9	81.4	78.2	80.9

The composition of the body fluids in childhood is also discussed by Josephson.[17]

Discussion

Interfering factors in flame photometry and precautions necessary for accurate emission spectrophotometry have been well summarized by Teloh.[1] Of course the interference effects vary with the different types of commercial instruments, depending upon the type of burner system, the fuel used, flame temperature, solvents, viscosity, optical systems, and the size of the slit width. Fortunately for sodium and potassium analysis, the nonspecific increase in flame background does not present as much of a problem as in the analysis of calcium, where blank solutions having concentrations of the elements approximately the same as that of the serum are frequently used to provide a uniform background. Many of the interference effects are eliminated by the use of the double photocell instrument.

Where the prism type of optical system is used, it is desirable to use as small a slit width as possible. The spectral light passed through the prism is proportional to the slit width, while the background and scattered radiations are proportional to the square of the slit width. Some instruments are equipped with a photomultiplier to permit use of narrower slit widths. Increasing the flame temperature also increases the intensity of background and scattered radiation.

In order to measure sodium and potassium levels reliably, especially with limited serum samples available, thorough familiarity with the instrument to be used and its limitations are most important. Distilled water should always be used, and polyethylene storage bottles are recommended to eliminate the leaching effect which significantly increases the sodium concentration of water stored in soft glass containers. As in other ultramicro determinations, evaporation should be carefully avoided. Pipets should be calibrated and kept chemically clean. Tobacco smoke, which contains considerable potassium, will adversely affect the accuracy of open aspirator systems using compressed atmospheric air to nebulize the sample. Smoking should not be permitted in the vicinity of the flame photometry. Fluctuations in gas pressure will affect readings; use of a booster pump is recommended with the Coleman instrument if gas pressure is under 5 inches of water or is unsteady. The rate of aspiration is very critical and the stylet should be used frequently to keep the atomizer from blocking. Highest accuracy is achieved by making several readings in rapid succession under identical conditions. (See section on calibration and control.)

Extreme caution must be exercised to avoid contamination. Separate test tubes and pipets should be reserved for use in this test only. Chromic acid cleaning solution (not detergents) should be used for cleaning glassware. Rubber stoppers should be avoided if possible, but if they are used they should be rinsed several times in distilled water and handled with clean forceps or crucible tongs. Care should be taken to avoid touching the rim of the test tubes with the fingers since this will result in sodium contamination. Contamination from tissue fluid in the collection of the specimen will give false low results. Hemolysis must be avoided since the high concentration of potassium in red blood cells will give an elevated serum level. High potassium levels may also result from refrigeration of clotted blood for even a few hours at 4 C.[2] When using plasma one should be sure that the anticoagulant does not contain potassium or sodium.

Smaller amounts of serum may be used if necessary to determine potassium. The following table shows the appropriate dilutions:

Microliters of serum	ml./Li solution	Dilution
25	2	1:80
50	3	1:60
75	5	1:66.7
100	5	1:50

Sodium is the primary determinant of tonicity in extracellular fluid. In diabetic ketosis, the increased blood sugar may add significantly to the osmolarity of extracellular fluid and consequently reduce serum sodium. Studies on experimental salt depletion[3] have shown that severe depletion is required before reduced levels of sodium are found. Clinical salt depletion therefore is primarily due to body losses rather than to dietary depletion. Losses from the gastrointestinal tract are common and excess sweating and urine sodium loss may also contribute. Renal failure, adrenal insufficiency, use of diuretics, chronic uremia, and salt-losing nephritis all cause urine sodium loss. Hyponatremia may also be induced by too vigorous sodium depletion during edema. This is especially true in congestive heart failure.[4]

All cases of sodium loss must be evaluated with reference to degree of hydration in which the primary abnormality is water retention.[5] In these conditions the sodium will revert to normal when the primary condition is brought under control. An increase of sodium concentration is less common. High serum sodium with low urine sodium has been found after head injury,[6] extracerebral neoplasm,[7] and other conditions involving the depression of consciousness.[8]

If the serum sodium is not readily obtainable or if a rough check on the accuracy of the determination is desirable, it may be roughly estimated by adding 10 to the sum of chloride and bicarbonate ion values expressed in mEq. The figure 10 must be increased in cases of diabetes or starvation (ketone bodies) and in nephritis (phosphate retention).

Sodium analysis of sweat has assumed considerable importance in the diagnosis of cystic fibrosis of the pancreas. Barbero[9] has summarized the results in the literature concerning concentrations of sodium in sweat of infants and children:

	Range	Mean
Control (351)	1.0-120 mEq./L.	28.1 mEq./L.
Cystic fibrosis (228)	36.4-215.4 mEq./L.	117.9 mEq./L.

In adults Peterson found mean sodium concentration in 262 persons to be 39.3 mEq./L., while sweat sodium concentration in patients with pulmonary diseases were 61.5 mEq./L.[10]

Normal potassium values vary more than sodium since the homeostatic mechanism is less efficient. In dietary potassium depletion, serum potassium may drop to low levels, but seldom less than 3.0 mEq./L. The comparatively large cellular reserves prevent further losses. Uncomplicated potassium depletion may be caused by sodium retention increasing the extracellular sodium, and with the development of extracellular alkalosis.[11] The alkalosis appears independent of any renal influence and is secondary to passage of Na^+ and H^- ions from extracellular to the intracellular compartment. The increase of serum bicarbonate and pH in potassium deficiency therefore indicates no gain of alkali or loss of acid from the body.

Low potassium levels usually, but not always, indicate potassium depletion. Depletion may occur without significant alterations in the serum potassium concentration, such as in diabetic ketosis and abnormal loss from the gastrointestinal tract. If the sodium depletion in the cases is corrected, low levels of potassium may be found.

Hypokalemia, like hyponatremia, is most often found when the ion is lost in gastrointestinal secretions or in urine. Vomiting will cause greater loss of potassium, since gastric juice has a high potassium content.

The kidney does not conserve potassium as well as sodium. Higher potassium levels are less common since the kidney efficiently excretes this ion. Renal failure may produce a definite hyperkalemia. High serum potassium may also be found in Addisonian crises.

Sodium and potassium levels in full-term and healthy premature infants are discussed by Natelson, Crawford and Munsey.[12] There is a slight transient rise in sodium during the first few days of life, the sodium level stabilizing at approximately 136 mEq./L. in the normal infant and 134 mEq./L. in the premature. During the period of physiologic jaundice, the potassium levels in the normal infant run rather high, frequently rising above 6 mEq./L. After 10 days, the level remains approximately 4.3 mEq./L. The potassium level of the healthy premature infant remains elevated during the more prolonged period of physiologic jaundice. This elevated potassium level after physiologic icterus has disappeared is considered to be of diagnostic significance in evaluation of so-called "adrenal immaturity."

Electrolyte management is frequently a problem in the premature infant and ultramicro chemistry plays an important role. Butterfield et al. present a study of electrolyte and nitrogen balance in the newborn premature infant.[13]

Circuit modifications have been described for the Model DB-2 Baird flame photometer to increase the ease of calibration and to enable sodium and potassium to be determined on the same sample dilution.[14] A further modification provides a three-channel circuit for measurement of both sodium and potassium without resetting controls.[15]

REFERENCES

1. Teloh, H. A.: Clinical Flame Photometry. Springfield, Ill., Charles C Thomas, 1959.
2. Goodman, J. R., Vincent, J., and Rosen, I.: Am. J. Clin. Path. 24: 111, 1954.
3. McCance, R. A.: Lancet 1: 823, 1936.
4. Schroeder, H. A.: J.A.M.A. 141: 117, 1949.
5. MacDonald, R. P.: J. Michigan M. Soc. 55: 538, 1956.
6. Higgins, G., Lewin, W., O'Brien, J. R. P., and Taylor, W. H.: Lancet 1: 1295, 1951.
7. Cooper, I. S., and Crevier P. H.: J. Clin. Endocrinol. 12: 821, 1952.
8. Zimmerman, B., and Freier, E. F.: Surgery 31: 373, 1952.
9. Barbero, G. J.: Pediatrics 24: 658, 1959.
10. Peterson, E. M.: J. A. M. A. 171: 87, 1959.
11. Wooton, I. D. P., Milne, M. D., and King, E. J.: Ann. Rev. Biochem. 23: 432, 1954.
12. Natelson, S., Crawford, W. L., and Munsey, F. A.: Correlation of Clinical and Chemical Observations in the Immature Infant. Richmond Hill, N. Y., Endo Products, Inc., 1952.
13. Butterfield, J., Lubchenco, L. O., Bergstedt, J., and O'Brien, D.: Pediatrics 26: 777, 1960.
14. MacDuffee, R. C.: Clin. Chem. 5: 492, 1959.

15. RAYMOND, S.: *Clin. Chem. 6:* 598, 1960.
16. GYLLENSWÄRD, C., AND JOSEPHSON, B.: *Scandinav. J. Clin. & Lab. Invest. 9:* 21, 1957.
17. JOSEPHSON, B.: Composition of the body fluids in childhood. *In* Advances in Clinical Chemistry, Vol. 1. New York, Academic Press, 1958.

23

Sulfanilamides

Principle

This is a modification of the Bratton-Marshall[1] method of determining blood sulfanilamide levels. The free primary aryl group of the sulfonamide is diazotized with nitrous acid and the excess nitrite destroyed with ammonium sulfamate. The diazotized sulfonamide is coupled with N-1-naphthyl)-ethylenediamine dihydrochloride to form a purplish-red azo dye.[2]

Apparatus

Pipets, KMP or other ultramicro type, 25, 200, 250 lambdas.
Centrifuge tubes, 1 ml.
Beckman DU spectrophotometer.

Reagents

1. *Trichloroacetic acid, 10 per cent:* Dilute 10 ml. concentrated trichloroacetic acid to 100 ml. with distilled water. Keeps about 1 month in a pyrex glass-stoppered bottle.

2. *Sodium nitrite, 0.5 per cent:* Dilute 5 ml. of 10 per cent sodium nitrite to 100 ml. with distilled water. Prepare as required for immediate use.

3. *Sodium nitrite, 10 per cent:* Dissolve 10 Gm. reagent quality sodium nitrite in distilled water and dilute to 100 ml. Keep in refrigerator.

4. *Ammonium sulfamate, 1.0 per cent:* Dissolve 1.0 Gm. ammonium sulfamate ($NH_2SO_3NH_4$) in distilled water and dilute to 100 ml. Discard if mold appears.

5. *N-(1-naphthyl)-ethylenediamine dihydrochloride, 0.2 per cent:* Dissolve 200 mg. N-(1-naphthyl)-ethylenediamine dihydrochloride ($C_{10}H_7NHCH_2CH_2NH_2 \cdot 2HCl$, EK4835) in 100 ml. distilled water. Keeps about one month in a brown bottle if refrigerated. Discard when brown color appears.

Procedure

1.   Transfer 25 lambdas serum to a 1 ml. centrifuge tube and 25 lambdas distilled water to another tube for a reagent blank. Add 500 lambdas of 10 per cent trichloroacetic acid, mix well, allow to stand for about 2 minutes, and centrifuge.

2.   Transfer 100 lambdas of the supernatant to a 13 × 100 mm. test tube. Add 200 lambdas of distilled water, 50 lambdas of 0.5 per cent sodium nitrite solution, mix well, and allow to stand for 3 minutes out of direct sunlight.[1]

3.   Add 100 lambas of 1 per cent ammonium sulfamate, mix and allow to stand 3 minutes.

4.   Add 100 lambdas of 0.2 per cent N-(1-naphthyl)-ethylenediamine dihydrochloride, and shake vigorously to dispel air bubbles. Avoid exposure to sunlight.[3] Let stand for 10 minutes.

5.   Transfer to ultramicro cuvets and read the optical density of the solution in a Beckman DU spectrophotometer at 540 mμ. Set at 100 per cent transmittance with distilled water; 10 per cent trichloroacetic acid is used as a blank. The result in mg. sulfanilamide per 100 ml. serum is determined by reference to a calibration curve.

Calibration

The calibration curve is prepared by diluting stock sulfanilamide standard solution (Harleco No. 29461, 1 ml. = 0.2 mg.) 1:10 with 10 per cent trichloroacetic acid and making up the following samples:

ml. Dilute standard	ml. 10 per cent TCA	Equivalent mg./100 ml. sulfa
0	10	0
1	9	4.2
2	8	8.4
3	7	12.6
4	6	16.8
5	5	21.0
6	4	25.2
7	3	29.4
8	2	33.6
9	1	37.8
10	0	42.0

For maximum precision the standard should contain the sulfa being measured.

A 100-lambda aliquot of the above samples is placed in a 13 × 100 mm. test tube and the sulfanilamide level determined as described above. Optical density is plotted against concentration for the calibration curve. The color developed conforms to Beer's law and the graph will be linear.

The standard solutions must be prepared in 10 per cent trichloroacetic acid. Alteration of the pH of the final solution will prevent color formation. A reagent blank should be run for each determination. The blank value will rise as the reagents age, but the difference of standard minus blank value will remain constant.

Results

This modification gives results which compare with the macro technic. If the type of sulfonamide being administered is unknown or if a combination of several sulfa drugs is being used, the value may be reported as "mg. per 100 ml. expressed as sulfanimilamide." If it is known, the value is obtained for sulfanilamide and converted to the appropriate sulfonamide by use of Table 10.

TABLE 10.

To express as	Multiply by
Sulfacetimide	1.24
Sulfadiazine	1.45
Sulfaguanidine	1.24
Sulfamerazine	1.53
Sulfamethyl-thiazole	1.56
Sulfanilyl-sulfanilamide	1.90
Sulfapyrazine	1.45
Sulfapyridine	1.45
Sulfasuxidine	2.06
Sulfathiazole	1.48
Gantrisin	2.26

Discussion

The small quantity of blood required for this determination permits the clinician to follow the blood level in infants during the course of sulfa therapy. Blood levels usually adequate to suppress susceptible organisms are approximately 10 to 15 mg. per 100 ml. for sulfadiazine and sulfamerazine in severe infections, 6 to 10 mg. per 100 ml. for moderate infections, and 2 to 3 mg. per 100 ml. for prophylaxis.[4, 5] Toxic reactions are frequent at higher blood levels. The level in the cerebrospinal fluid varies from 20 to 100 per cent that of the blood, depending on the sulfonamide used and its permeability.

REFERENCES

1. BRATTON, C. A., AND MARSHALL, E. K., JR.: *J. Biol. Chem. 128:* 537, 1939.
2. MACDONALD, R. P., AND PLOOMPUU, J.: *Mikrochim. Acta 147,* 1958.
3. HELBOURN, A. H. S., AND PATTLE, R. E.: *J. Lab. & Clin. Med. 28:* 1028, 1943.
4. CLARKE, G. H.: *Am. J. Dis. Child. 73:* 565, 1947.
5. WOLMAN, I. J.: Laboratory Applications in Clinical Pediatrics. New York, McGraw-Hill, 1957.

24

Thymol Turbidity

Principle

A saturated solution of thymol in barbital buffer of pH 7.55 produces turbidity in serum from patients with liver disease. Barium sulfate standards of known concentration are used to compare turbidity and the result is expressed in arbitrary units.

Apparatus

Pipet, KMP or other ultramicro type, 10 lambdas
Pipet, Mohr, 1.0 ml.
Test tubes, 13 × 100 mm.

Reagents

1. *Thymol buffer reagent, pH 7.55:* Place in a one-liter pyrex beaker 1.00 Gm. sodium barbital N.F. (Veronal), 1.50 Gm. barbituric acid (Barbital) and 3.0 Gm. of high quality thymol crystals. Add 500 ml. of distilled water and bring to a boil with occasional stirring. Cool to room temperature, cover and allow to stand overnight. Seed with a few thymol crystals to remove supersaturation, mix and allow to stand 30 minutes. Filter into a clean glass-stoppered brown bottle. If possible, check on a pH meter. This solution will keep several weeks at room temperature. Do not refrigerate, and discard the solution if it becomes cloudy.

2. *Barium chloride, 0.0962N:* Transfer 1.175 Gm. reagent quality barium chloride ($BaCl_2:2H_2O$) to a 100 ml. volumetric flask. Dissolve in about 50 ml. of distilled water, dilute to mark and mix.

3. *Sulfuric acid, 0.2N:* Measure about 800 ml. of distilled water into a one liter volumetric flask. Add *carefully* 5.6 ml. of concentrated reagent quality sulfuric acid, mix and dilute to mark and mix again. Cool before using.

Procedure

    1.   **Pipet 0.60 ml. thymol buffer reagent into 13 × 100 mm. test tube.**

    2.   *Add* **10 lambdas of serum.**

    3.   **Mix and allow to stand at room temperature for *30 minutes*.**

    4.   **Read the optical density in a Beckman DU spectrophotometer at 660 mμ using distilled water to set the instrument at 100 per cent transmittance.**

Calculation

    OD sample × F = thymol turbidity in units.

        See *Calibration* for Factor (F)

Calibration

    1. Transfer 0.5, 1.0, 2.0, 3.0, 4.0 and 5.0 ml. of barium chloride solution into separate 100 ml. volumetric flasks. Dilute to mark with 0.2N sulfuric acid at 10 C. and mix thoroughly.

    2. Optical density of these suspensions should be read *within 5-10 minutes* in a Beckman DU spectrophotometer at 660 mμ using distilled water to set the instrument at 100 per cent transmittance.

    3. In the method described, these standards correspond to a thymol turbidity of 3.7, 7.4, 14.8, 22.2, 29.6 and 37 units.

$$F = \frac{\text{equivalent units}}{\text{OD of standard}}$$

    A calibration curve should be plotted to determine the extent of linearity. The mean of the F values may be used for calculating daily determinations. This method will give results agreeing with the Shank-Hoagland macro technic.[1] To convert to Maclagan units, divide the Shank-Hoagland units by two.

Normal Values

    0-4 units.

Discussion

    The thymol turbidity test of Maclagan[2-5] is based on the appearance of turbidity when serum from patients with hepatocellular damage is added to a saturated solution of thymol in barbital buffer. The exact mechanism for the turbidity formation is in dispute. The reagent reacts with proteins, lipids and lipoproteins, and blood must be obtained from fasting patients since lipemia will increase the thymol turbidity values.[6-11] Investigators have reported the principal reactant to be beta-globulin,[12-13] gamma-globulin,[3, 14-17] or both beta- and gamma-globulins.[6, 18-20]

Considerable confusion has resulted in attempts to interpret and compare results of this test; not only because of the conflicting Maclagan-Shank-Hoagland units, but because of the introduction of a more sensitive buffering system,[21] the various modifications of the thymol barbital reagent, [22-23] and the fundamental differences in optical characteristics of the photometers used.[8, 24]

In spite of this, thymol turbidity is among the most useful of liver function tests. It is often elevated in viral hepatitis and may be used to determine the degree of recovery of the patient. It has proved especially helpful in blood donor screening by detecting at least some of the subclinical carriers of virus hepatitis.[25-28] In early biliary obstruction, the thymol turbidity is usually within normal limits but prolonged obstruction, with its resultant damage to the hepatic parenchyma, will occasionally cause the thymol turbidity to become elevated. The complexity of the reaction in these patients, with interference by the bile salt-phospholipid-cholesterol complex and serum mucoproteins, is discussed by Ducci.[29]

If the serum to be used for this test must be stored before analysis, Yonan and Reinhold recommend that it be allowed to remain in contact with the cells.[34] Decreased values will occur if the serum is separated from the cells prior to storage.

In general, thymol turbidity is elevated in diseases where increases in gamma-globulin occur. These include tuberculosis, sarcoidosis, multiple myeloma, lymphogranuloma, lupus erythematosis and hypersensitivity reactions. Thymol turbidity is reported to be lower in infants than in adults,[30] and is not considered reliable in infants under six months.[31] Serial bilirubin tests are considered more reliable for this group.[32] A fine review of the thymol test and the factors affecting its accuracy is presented in articles by Reinhold and Yonan.[33, 34]

REFERENCES

1. SHANK, R. E., AND HOAGLAND, C. L.: *J. Biol. Chem. 162:* 133, 1946.
2. MACLAGAN, N. F.: *Brit. J. Exper. Path. 25:* 234, 1944.
3. ————, AND BUNN, D.: *Biochem. J. 41:* 580, 1947.
4. ————: *Brit. M. J. 2:* 197, 1947.
5. ————, MARTIN, N. H., AND LUNNON, J. G.: *J. Clin. Path. 5:* 1, 1952.
6. KUNKEL, H. G., AND HOAGLAND, C. L.: *J. Clin. Invest. 26:* 1060, 1947.
7. REINHOLD, J. G.: *Clin. Chem. 1:* 3, 1955.
8. ————: *Clin. Chem. 1:* 351, 1955.

9. SHAY, H., BERK, J. E., AND SIPLET, H.: *Gastroenterology 9*: 644, 1947.
10. POPPER, H., STEIGMAN, F., DYNIEWIZ, H., AND DUBIN, A.: *J. Lab. & Clin. Med. 33*: 1630, 1948.
11. KATZ, E. J., HASTERLIK, R. J., AND SNAPP, F. E.: *J. Lab. & Clin. Med. 44*: 353, 1954.
12. COHEN, P. P., AND THOMPSON, F. L.: *J. Lab. & Clin. Med. 32*: 475, 1947.
13. REGANT, L.: *J. Lab. & Clin. Med. 44*: 917, 1954.
14. RALLI, E. P., LESLIE, S. H., STUCK, G. H., JR., SHORR, H. E., ROBSON, J. S., CLARKE, D. H., AND LAKEN, B.: *Medicine 28*: 301, 1949.
15. HAVENS, W. P., JR., AND WILLIAMS, T. L.: *Acta med. scandinav. Suppl. 136*: 141, 1949.
16. MARRACK, J. R., JOHNS, R. G. S., AND HOCH, H.: *Brit. J. Exper. Path. 31*: 36, 1950.
17. KIBRICK, A. C., RODGERS, H. E., AND SKUPP, S. J.: *Am. J. Clin. Path. 22*: 698, 1952.
18. MARTIN, N. H.: *J. Am. Chem. Soc. 71*: 1230, 1949.
19. _____: *J. Clin. Path. 2*: 275, 1949.
20. ALBERTSEN, K., CHRISTOFFERSEN, N. R., AND HEINTZELMANN, F.: *Acta med. scandinav. 136*: 302, 1950.
21. MATEER, J. G., BALTZ, J. I., COMANDURAS, P. D., STEEL, H. H., BROWER, S. W., AND YAGLE, E. M.: *Gastroenterology 8*: 52, 1947.
22. DE LA HUERGA, H., AND POPPER, H.: *J. Lab. & Clin. Med. 34*: 877, 1949.
23. YONAN, V. L., AND REINHOLD, J. G.: *Am. J. Clin. Path. 24*: 232, 1954.
24. HOYER, G., AND JORGENSEN, J.: *Scandinav. J. Clin. & Lab. Invest. 4*: 319, 1952.
25. NEEFE, J. R., NORRIS, R. F., REINHOLD, J. G., MITCHELL, C. B., AND HOWELL, E. S.: *J.A.M.A. 154*: 1066, 1954.
26. JENNINGS, E. R.: Personal communication.
27. FITCH, D. R., WATANABE, R. K., KASSOUNY, D., NEEFE, J. R., REINHOLD, J. G., AND NORRIS, R. F.: *Am. J. Clin. Path. 25*: 158, 1955.
28. NEEFE, J. R.: *In* SCHIFF, L.: Diseases of the Liver. Philadelphia, Lippincott, 1956.
29. DUCCI, H.: *In* SHERLOCK, S., AND WOLSTENHOLME, G. E. W., Liver Disease. Philadelphia, Blakiston, 1951.
30. DESMOND, M. M., ZIMMERMAN, H. J., SWEET, L. K., AND THOMAS, L. J.: *Pediatrics 3*: 49, 1949.
31. GELLIS, S. S., AND HSIA, D. Y. Y.: *New England J. Med. 249*: 400, 1953.
32. HSIA, D. Y. Y., AND GELLIS, S. S.: *Am. J. Dis. Child. 85*: 13, 1953.
33. REINHOLD, J. G., AND YONAN, V. L.: *Am. J. Clin. Path. 26*: 669, 1956.
34. YONAN, V. L., AND REINHOLD, J. G.: *Clin. Chem. 3*: 685, 1957.

25

Urea Nitrogen

Principle

This is an ultramicro adaptation of the Fearon[1] diacetyl monoxime method as modified by Friedman.[2] The urea in a protein free filtrate is heated with diacetyl monoxime and the color developed by treatment with arsenic-sulfuric acid reagent. The acid reagent oxidizes the hydroxylamine formed since the latter would otherwise inhibit color development.

Apparatus

Pipet, KMP or other ultramicro type, 25 lambdas (2)
Pipet, KMP or other ultramicro type, 50 lambdas (2)
Pipet, KMP or other ultramicro type, 100 lambdas
Pipet, KMP or other ultramicro type, 250 lambdas
Centrifuge tubes, micro, 1.0 ml.
Test tubes, 7 × 70 mm.

Reagents

1. *Trichloroacetic acid, conc.:* Dissolve 100 Gm. reagent quality crystalline trichloroacetic acid in distilled water and dilute to 100 ml. This reagent will keep indefinitely if stored in a pyrex glass-stoppered bottle.

2. *Trichloroacetic acid, 10 per cent:* Dilute 10 ml. of concentrated trichloroacetic acid to 100 ml. with distilled water and store in a glass-stoppered pyrex bottle. Prepare fresh each week.

3. *Diacetyl monoxime, 1 per cent:* Dissolve 1 Gm. of diacetyl monoxime (Eastman) in 100 ml. of 5 per cent reagent quality acetic acid.

4. *Arsenic-sulfuric acid:* By careful stirring and cooling, add 50 ml. of concentrated reagent quality sulfuric acid to 50 ml. of distilled water in a 250 ml. Erlenmeyer flask. After cooling the mixture to about 50 C., add 10 Gm. of reagent quality arsenic acid (H_3AsO_4), mix well and allow to cool. Store in a glass-stoppered pyrex bottle.

5. *Urea stock standard solution:* Transfer 0.5359 Gm. of dry reagent quality urea to a 500 ml. volumetric flask. Dissolve in distilled water and dilute to mark and mix. The solution is equivalent to a concentration of 50 mg. urea N per 100 ml. of serum.

Procedure

1.　Transfer 25 lambdas of serum to a one ml. centrifuge tube.

2.　Add 250 lambdas of distilled water and 250 lambdas of 10 per cent trichloroacetic acid. Mix solution thoroughly and centrifuge for 10 minutes in an ultramicro centrifuge.

3.　Transfer 100 lambdas of clear supernatant solution to a 7 x 70 mm. test tube. Prepare a reagent blank by transferring 100 lambdas of distilled water to another 7 x 70 mm. test tube. Add 50 lambdas of diacetyl monoxime reagent to each tube and mix thoroughly.

4.　Add 100 lambdas of arsenic-sulfuric acid reagent, mix by gently tapping and place in a boiling water bath for exactly 10 minutes.

5.　Remove and allow to cool at room temperature for exactly 3 minutes. Add 250 lambdas of distilled water, mix and transfer to an ultramicro cuvette.

6.　Read the optical density of the unknown and blank solutions within 10 minutes in a Beckman spectrophotometer at 475 mμ using distilled water to set the instrument at 100 per cent transmittance.

7.　If the absorbence of the unknown is greater than that previously determined for 50 mg. per cent, the colored solution should be diluted with an equal volume of distilled water and the final result multiplied by two. If necessary, the dilution step may be repeated but caution should be taken to insure that the reading is done within the 10-minute time interval.

Calculations

The optical density of the reagent blank is subtracted from the optical density of the unknown and the value of urea nitrogen in mg. per 100 ml obtained directly from the calibration curve. The use of a factor is not advised since the calibration curve is not a straight line.

Calibration

1. Prepare two working standard solutions as follows:

(a) 1 mg. per cent urea N: Pipet 2 ml. of stock standard solution into a 100 ml. volumetric flask, dilute to mark with distilled water and mix;

(b) 5 mg. per cent urea N: Pipet 10 ml. of stock standard solution into a 100 ml. volumetric flask, dilute to mark with distilled water and mix. These two solutions are diluted as follows to prepare a calibration curve.

ml. working standard	ml. distilled water	Eq. mg/100 ml. Urea N
1A	9	2.1
2A	8	4.2
3A	7	6.3
5A	5	10.5
7A	3	14.7
10A	0	21.0
3B	7	31.5
4B	6	42.0
5B	5	52.5
7B	3	73.5
10B	0	105.0

2. Place 100 lambdas of each dilute standard in a 7 x 70 mm. test tube.

3. Add 50 lambdas of diacetyl monoxime and 100 lambdas of arsenic-sulfuric acid reagent to each tube.

4. Continue as described under *Procedure*.

5. Plot the optical density against equivalent serum urea nitrogen concentration on a sheet of graph paper. The curve will not be an absolutely straight line, especially above 50 mg. per 100 ml. concentration. It is best to dilute the final colored solution so that the result may be measured between the 10 and 50 mg. per 100 ml. area on the graph. The blank need not be diluted with the unknown since no appreciable error will be introduced by omitting this step.

Normal Values

10-20 mg. per 100 ml. of serum.

Discussion

This method shows good agreement with the Karr urease method of determining blood urea nitrogen. The slight inaccuracies introduced by dilution at high levels are of no clinical significance. This method does not produce the strong odors found objectionable in other methods, i.e., free diacetyl[3] or fuming hydrochloric acid.[4] Adaptations of the method of Fearon[1] and Friedman[2] are included in both the Spinco and Coleman ultramicro systems.

Blood should be obtained while the patient is in a fasting state as higher levels occur following meals, especially if they are rich in protein. Urea nitrogen is elevated in a large number of disease states and the cause may be either of renal or extrarenal origin. This subject is fully discussed in clinical pathology texts. The ultramicro method finds its greatest use in postoperative patients and severe burn cases.

UREASE METHOD

Principle

The urea in serum is hydrolyzed to ammonium carbonate by direct incubation with glycerol urease. Proteins are precipitated with tungstic acid and a portion of the protein free supernatant is subjected to Nesslerization and compared photometrically with a standard urea solution which is treated similarly.

Apparatus

Pipets, KMP or other ultramicro type, 10 lambdas (1)
Pipets, KMP or other ultramicro type, 25 lambdas (2)
Pipets, KMP or other ultramicro type, 100 lambdas (2)
Pipets, KMP or other ultramicro type, 200 lambdas (2)
Micro test tubes, 1 ml.
Microcentrifuge tubes, 1 ml.

Reagents

1. *Glycerol urease:*   Harleco Item #3028.
2. *Tungstic acid* deproteinizing reagent (same as for glucose method).
3. *Nessler's reagent:* Commercially made reagent should be purchased (Koch-McMeekin formula).
4. *Iodine solution, 0.5 per cent:*   Dissolve 0.45 Gm. of potassium iodide and 0.50 Gm. of iodine crystals in 5 ml. of water and dilute to 100 ml. Store in glass-stoppered brown bottle.
5. *Stock urea nitrogen standard* (100 mg./100 ml.):   Dissolve 2.144 Gm. desiccator-dried urea in water and dilute to 1 liter.

Procedure

1. Pipet 25 lambdas serum into 1 ml. centrifuge tube.
2. Add 100 lambdas distilled water.
3. Add 25 lambdas of glycerol urease, mix well, stopper and let stand at room temperature for 15 minutes.
4. Add 400 lambdas protein precipitating reagent, mix, and centrifuge for 2-3 minutes in an ultramicro centrifuge.
5. Pipet 200 lambdas clear supernatant into a one ml. micro test tube.
6. Add 250 lambdas distilled water; mix.
7. Add 10 lambdas iodine solution.
8. Add 100 lambdas Nessler's reagent and mix.
9. Read in Beckman DU at 480 mμ.

Blank: Use 25 lambdas of distilled water instead of serum.

Standard: Use 25 lambdas of a suitable urea nitrogen standard.

Calculation

$$\frac{\text{mg./100 ml. urea N in standard} \times (\text{O.D. unknown—O.D. blank})}{\text{O.D. standard—O.D. blank}} = \begin{array}{l}\text{mg./100 ml.}\\ \text{urea N in}\\ \text{unknown}\end{array}$$

Calibration

A calibration curve should be made to determine the extent of its linearity. Dilute stock urea N standard (100 mg./100 ml.) 5 to 100.

Prepare calibration standards as follows:

Amount of diluted standard	Amount of H$_2$O	Corresponding value
1 ml.	9 ml.	11.0 mg./100 ml.
2	8	22.0
3	7	33.0
4	6	44.0
5	5	55.0
6	4	66.0
7	3	77.0
8	2	88.0
9	1	99.0
10	0	110.0

Use calibration standards as 200 lambdas protein-free filtrate in step 6 in method.

The corresponding value of the calibration standards is based on the 1:22 dilution of the serum in the method.

Normal Values

10-20 mg. per 100 ml. of serum.

Discussion

Many laboratories use a urease method for macro urea nitrogen studies and would prefer to use a similar ultramicro procedure. This method gives good reproducibility and has been found to be accurate to within ± 4 per cent. Recovery studies on four known specimens showed the following per cent recovered: 103.4 per cent, 98.4 per cent, 96.2 per cent, and 99.0 per cent.

If Lab-Trol is used as a standard for this method, the pH of the Lab-Trol protein-free standard must be raised just before adding urease; otherwise the conversion of urea to ammonium carbonate will be incomplete and values will be low because of the slowness of the reaction. 0.1 N NaOH is added to the Lab-Trol protein free standard in the proportion of 80 lambdas per 500 lambdas of standard.

REFERENCES

Diacetyl Monoxime Method
1. FEARON, W. R.: *Biochem. J. 33:* 902, 1939.
2. FRIEDMAN, H. S.: *Anal. Chem. 25:* 662, 1953.
3. NATELSON, S., SCOTT, M. L., AND BEFFE, C.: *Am. J. Clin. Path. 21:* 275, 1951.
4. KAMERAU, E.: *Sci. Proc. Roy. Dublin Soc. 42:* 63, 1946.
5. SKEGGS, L. T.: *Am. J. Clin. Path. 28:* 311, 1957.
6. MARSH, W. H., FINGERHUT, B., AND KIRSCH, E.: *Am. J. Clin. Path. 28:* 681, 1957.
7. RICHTER, H. J., AND LAPOINTE, Y. S.: *Clin. Chem. 5:* 617, 1959.

Urease Method
8. VAN SLYKE, D. D., AND CULLEN, G. E.: *J. Biol. Chem. 24:* 117, 1916.
9. KARR, W. B.: *J. Lab. & Clin. Med. 9:* 329, 1924.
10. MACFATE, R. P., COHN, C., EICHELBERGER, L., AND COOPER, J. A. D.: *Am. J. Clin Path. 24:* 511, 1954.
11. GENZKOW, C. J.: *J. Biol. Chem. 149:* 255, 1943.
12. NELSON, N.: *J. Biol. Chem. 153:* 375, 1944.
13. ANNINO, J. S.: Clinical Chemistry. New York, Little Brown & Co., 1956.
14. CONNERTY, H. V., BRIGGS, A. R., AND EATON, E. H.: *Am. J. Clin. Path. 25:* 1321, 1955.
15. KING, J. W., AND FAULKNER, W. R.: Workshop on Microchemistry, Pre-Workshop and Technique Manuals. Chicago, Am. Soc. Clin. Path., 1960.

16. CONWAY, E. J.: Microdiffusion Analysis and Volumetric Error, 4th ed. London, C. Lockwood & Son, Ltd., 1957.
17. SELIGSON, D., AND HIRAHARA, K.: *J. Lab. & Clin. Med. 49:* 962, 1957.

Alpha-Isonitrosopropiophenone Method

18. MEITES, S.: Laboratory Manual of Clinical Chemistry. Columbus, Ohio, The Children's Hospital of Columbus, 1959.
19. —————, AND FAULKNER, W. R.: Manual of Practical Micro and General Procedures in Clinical Chemistry. Springfield, Ill., Charles C Thomas, 1962.

26

Uric Acid

Principle

A Folin-Wu protein-free filtrate is used to determine uric acid. The uric acid reacts with phosphotungstic acid to form a blue color. In this technic sodium carbonate is used as the alkali instead of the more common sodium cyanide.[1, 2] While the cyanide provides increased sensitivity, this procedure is considered adequate for clinical purposes.

Apparatus

Pipet, KMP or other ultramicro type, 10 lambdas
Pipet, KMP or other ultramicro type, 20 lambdas
Pipet, KMP or other ultramicro type, 50 lambdas
Pipet, KMP or other ultramicro type, 100 lambdas
Pipet, 0.2 ml. serologic
Centrifuge tube, 1 ml. micro.
Test tubes, 7 x 70 mm.

Reagents

1. *Sulfuric acid, 2/3 N:* See under *Glucose.*
2. *Sodium tungstate, 10 per cent:* See under *Glucose.*
 (*Note:* Do *not* use pre-mixed Folin-Wu precipitating reagents.)
3. *Phosphotungstic acid reagent:*[2] Transfer 40 Gm. of sodium tungstate, $Na_2WO_4 \cdot 2H_2O$ to a one-liter boiling flask with a reflux condenser. Add 300 ml. of distilled water and swirl to dissolve the salt. Add 32 ml. of 85 per cent o-phosphoric acid and several glass beads. Reflux gently for 2 hours. Cool to room temperature and add water to a total volume of 1 liter. Add 32 Gm. of lithium sulfate, $Li_2SO_4 \cdot H_2O$, and mix to dissolve. This reagent is stable in a refrigerator.
4. *Sodium carbonate, 14 per cent:* Dissolve 14 Gm. of anhydrous sodium

carbonate in distilled water and dilute to 100 ml. Store in a polyethylene bottle.

5. *Stock uric acid standard, 1 mg. per ml.:* Weigh exactly 100 mg. of uric acid and 60 mg. of lithium carbonate, Li_2CO_3, and transfer to a 100 ml. volumetric flask. Add approximately 50 ml. of distilled water, and warm to approximately 60 C. in order to dissolve the ingredients. Cool to room temperature and dilute to mark with distilled water. This reagent is stable in a refrigerator.

6. *Working uric acid standard:* Dilute 0.5 ml. of stock standard to 50 ml. with distilled water. This is equivalent to a serum concentration of 10 mg. per cent uric acid. Prepare fresh daily.

Procedure

1. Pipet 160 lambdas of distilled water into a 1 ml. centrifuge tube. It is convenient to use a 0.2 ml. serologic pipet.

2. Add with rinsing 20 lambdas of serum.

3. Add 10 lambdas of 2/3 N sulfuric acid. Mix.

4. Add 10 lambdas of 10 per cent sodium tungstate. Mix well and centrifuge for 3-5 minutes.

5. Transfer 60 lambdas of filtrate, distilled water, and working standard to each of three 7 × 70 mm. test tubes. Label these tubes unknown, blank, and standard.

6. Add 20 lambdas of 14 per cent sodium carbonate. Mix.

7. Add 20 lambdas of phosphotungstic acid reagent. Mix, and allow to stand at room temperature for 15 minutes.

8. Add to each tube 100 lambdas of distilled water and mix.

9. Transfer to micro cuvets and read within 30 minutes in a spectrophotometer at 710 mμ wavelength, setting the instrument at 100 per cent transmittance with the reagent blank.

Calculation

$$\frac{OD_x}{OD_s} \times 10 = \text{mg. per 100 ml. uric acid}$$

or use calibration curve described below.

Calibration

1. *Working standard, 20 mg. per 100 ml.:* Dilute 1 ml. stock standard to 50 ml. with distilled water.

2. Prepare standards for a calibration curve by diluting this working stand-

ard 1.0, 2.0, 3.0, 5.0, 7.0 and 10.0 ml. to 10 ml. with distilled water using a 10 ml. volumetric flask. These standards are equivalent to 2, 4, 6, 10, 14, and 20 mg. per cent uric acid.

3. Proceed with step 5 under procedure.

4. Plot a calibration curve. The curve should be linear up to the 20 mg. per 100 ml. standard.

Normal Values

3-7 mg. per 100 ml.

Discussion

This procedure is an ultramicro modification of the macro method of Henry, Sobel and Kim.[2] The phosphotungstic acid reagent is a 2.5-fold dilution of that described by Folin and Denis,[3] with lithium sulfate added to suppress the formation of turbidity.[4] All reagents are used in the same proportion as the macro method. Use of "half quantities" of precipitating reagents results in a filtrate pH of 3.0-4.3. Good recovery of added uric acid is reported when the pH of the filtrate is above 3.0.[2]

The use of carbonate rather than cyanide has at least three advantages: (1) the reagent blanks are nearly colorless; (2) standard curves are very reproducible, and the precision of the method is excellent; (3) the poisonous properties of cyanide almost preclude its use in an ultramicro procedure.

Substances in serum other than uric acid account for approximately 11 per cent of the color produced by the phosphotungstate reaction.

The Coleman ultramicro analytical program utilizes Archibald's modification[5] of the method of Kern and Stransky,[6] also avoiding the use of sodium cyanide. Phosphotungstic acid is used both for the precipitation of proteins and the color development. O'Brien et al.[7] suggests that modifications of Caraway's procedure (also used in the Beckman/Spinco system) should include 5 per cent albumin in the standard solutions to restore linearity to the calibration curve.

REFERENCES

1. CARAWAY, W. T.: *Am. J. Clin Path.* 25: 840, 1955.
2. HENRY, R. J., SOBEL, C., AND KIM, J.: *Am. J. Clin. Path.* 28: 152, 1957.
3. FOLIN, O., AND DENIS, W.: *J. Biol. Chem.* 13: 469, 1912-13.
4. FOLIN, O.: *J. Biol. Chem.* 86: 179, 1930.
5. ARCHIBALD, R. M.: *Clin. Chem.* 3: 102, 1957.
6. KERN, A., AND STRANSKY, E.: *Biochem. Ztschr.* 290: 419, 1937.
7. O'BRIEN, D., IBBOTT, F., AND PINFIELD, A.: *Clin. Chem.* 7: 521, 1961.

Directory of Distributors and Producers

Advanced Instruments, Inc., 45 Kenneth St., Newton Highlands 61, Mass.

Allied Chemical and Dye Corp., General Chemical Division, 40 Rector Street, New York 6, N. Y.

American Hospital Supply Corp. (Scientific Products Div.), 1210 Leon Place, Evanston, Ill.

Baird-Atomic, Inc., 33 University Road, Cambridge 38, Mass.

Beckman Instruments, Inc., Scientific Instruments Division, 2500 Fullerton Road, Fullerton, Calif.

Beckman/Spinco Div., Stanford Industrial Park, Palo Alto, Calif.

Baltimore Biological Lab., Inc., 1460 Gorsuch, Avenue Baltimore 18, Md.

Bausch and Lomb Optical Co., 635 St. Paul Street, Rochester 2, N. Y.

Brinkmann Co., 115 Cutter Mill Rd., Great Neck, L. I., N. Y.

Chicago Apparatus Co., 1735 North Ashland Avenue, Chicago 22, Ill.

Clay-Adams, 141 East 25th St., New York 10, N. Y.

Coleman Instruments, Inc., 42 Madison St., Maywood, Ill.

College of American Pathologists, Prudential Plaza, Chicago 1, Ill.

Commercial Filters Corp., Melrose 76, Mass.

Consolidated Laboratories, Inc., P. O. Box 234, Chicago Heights, Ill.

Difco Laboratories, Inc., 920 Henry Street, Detroit, Mich.

Drummond Scientific Co., 524-526 N. 61st Street, Philadelphia 31, Pa.

Dynalab Corp., P.O. Box 112, Rochester 1, N. Y.

Eastman (Distillation Products Industries), Organic Chemicals Department, Rochester 3, N. Y.

Eberbach and Son Co., P.O. Box 63, Ann Arbor, Mich.

Fisher Scientific Co., 717 Forbes St., Pittsburgh, Pa.

Greiner Scientific Corp., Canal St. Station, Box 125L, N. Y. 13, N. Y.

Hartman-Leddon Co., 60th & Woodland Ave., Philadelphia 43, Pa.

International Equipment Co., 1284 Soldiers Field Rd., Boston 35, Mass.

K & K Laboratories, Inc., 177-10 93rd Ave., Jamaica 33, New York

Kimble Glass Co., P.O. Box 1035, Toledo 1, Ohio

Kopp and Staub Corp., 405 E. 62nd St., N. Y. 21, N. Y.

Labline, Inc., 3070-82 W. Grand Ave., Chicago 22, Ill.

The London Co., 3355 Edgecliff Terrace, Cleveland 11, Ohio

Manostat Corp., 20-26 N. Moore St., N. Y. 13, N. Y.

Mayer and Myles Laboratories, Allentown, Pa.

Microchemical Specialties Co., 1825 Eastshore Hwy., Berkeley 10, Calif.

Narda Ultrasonics Corp., 625 Main Street, Westbury, N. Y.

Nuclear Science Assoc., 56 Manor Dr., Newark 6, N. Y.

Photovolt Corp., 95 Madison Ave., N. Y. 16, N. Y.

Pyrocell Manufacturing Co., 207-11 E. 84th St., N. Y. 28, N. Y.

Quaracell Products Inc., 366 Broadway, N. Y. 13, N. Y.

Research Specialties Co., 200 South Garrard Blvd., Richmond, Calif.

Richard-Allan Co., Inc. 1335 Dodge Ave., Evanston, Ill.

Scientific Industries, Inc., 15 Park St., Springfield 3, Mass.

Scientific Service Laboratories, P.O. Box 175, Dallas 21, Texas

Sigma Chemical Co., 3500 DeKalb St., St. Louis 18, Mo.

Ivan Sorvall, Inc., Norwalk, Conn.

Sylvana Chemical Corp., Orange, N. J.

Takamine Laboratories, 1127 Myrtle, Elkhart, Ind.

Thermolyne Corp., 478 Huff St., Dubuque, Ia.

A. H. Thomas Co., West Washington Square, Philadelphia 5, Pa.

Warner-Chilcott, Division of Warner-Lambert, Pharmaceutical Company, Tabor Rd., Morris Plains, N. J.

West Co., West Bridge, Phoenixville, Pa.

Worthington Biochemical Co., Freehold, N. J.

Index